The
Hands-on Guide
to Practical Paediatrics

D1339412

To my family and friends and most of all to Nick, for your endless support, patience and encouragement.

Rebecca Hewitson

I would like to dedicate this book to my paediatric colleagues Heather Mackinnon and Mervyn Jaswon.

Caroline Fertleman

The
Hands-on Guide
to Practical Paediatrics

REBECCA HEWITSON
Paediatrics Specialist Trainee, London Deanery
The Whittington Hospital and Royal Free Hospital

CAROLINE FERTLEMAN
Consultant Paediatrician, The Whittington Hospital
Site Sub-Dean and Honorary Senior Lecturer,
University College London Medical School
Training Programme Director, School of Paediatrics, London Deanery
Honorary Consultant, Great Ormond Street Hospital, London

WILEY Blackwell

This edition first published 2014 © John Wiley & Sons, Ltd

Registered Office
John Wiley & Sons, Ltd, The Atrium, Southern Gate, Chichester, West Sussex, PO19 8SQ, UK

Editorial Offices
350 Main Street, Malden, MA 02148–5020, USA
9600 Garsington Road, Oxford, OX4 2DQ, UK
The Atrium, Southern Gate, Chichester, West Sussex, PO19 8SQ, UK

For details of our global editorial offices, for customer services, and for information about how to apply for permission to reuse the copyright material in this book please see our website at www.wiley.com/wiley-blackwell.

The right of Rebecca Hewitson and Caroline Fertleman to be identified as the authors of this work has been asserted in accordance with the UK Copyright, Designs and Patents Act 1988.

Wiley also publishes its books in a variety of electronic formats. Some content that appears in print may not be available in electronic books.

Designations used by companies to distinguish their products are often claimed as trademarks. All brand names and product names used in this book are trade names, service marks, trademarks or registered trademarks of their respective owners. The publisher is not associated with any product or vendor mentioned in this book.

Limit of Liability/Disclaimer of Warranty: While the publisher and author(s) have used their best efforts in preparing this book, they make no representations or warranties with respect to the accuracy or completeness of the contents of this book and specifically disclaim any implied warranties of merchantability or fitness for a particular purpose. It is sold on the understanding that the publisher is not engaged in rendering professional services and neither the publisher nor the author shall be liable for damages arising herefrom. If professional advice or other expert assistance is required, the services of a competent professional should be sought.

Library of Congress Cataloging-in-Publication Data

Hewitson, Rebecca, author.
  The hands-on guide to practical paediatrics / Rebecca Hewitson, Caroline Fertleman.
    p. ; cm.
  Includes bibliographical references and index.
  ISBN 978-1-118-46352-9 (paper. : alk. paper) – ISBN 978-1-118-46357-4 (eMobi) –
ISBN 978-1-118-46358-1 (ePub) – ISBN 978-1-118-46359-8 (ePDF) – ISBN 978-1-118-79386-2 –
ISBN 978-1-118-79408-1
  I. Fertleman, Caroline, author. II. Title.
  [DNLM: I. Pediatrics. WS 100]
  RJ61
  618.92–dc23

                                                    2013024995

A catalogue record for this book is available from the British Library.

Cover images: iStock photo, file #3313409, reproduced from iStock © slovegrove; iStock photo, file #18250395, reproduced from iStock © kajakiki; iStock photo, file #10579373, reproduced from iStock © yumiyum; iStock photo, file #1262714, reproduced from iStock © zoomstudio; iStock photo, file #11395745, reproduced from iStock © naumoid.
Cover design by Grounded Design

Set in 8/10pt Gill Sans by SPi Publisher Services, Pondicherry, India
Printed and bound in Malaysia by Vivar Printing Sdn Bhd

1 2014

Contents

5 Common paediatric emergencies

Preface

Working with children is enormously rewarding and varied but also has its own unique set of challenges. With most medical schools focusing predominantly on adult medicine, junior doctors can sometimes feel daunted by the prospect of interactions with younger patients and their families.

As part of the 'Hands on Guide' series, this book guides you through some of these challenges and acts as a companion for survival during daily clinical practice. We set out to write a book filled with practical advice in a concise and down-to-earth style and have avoided focusing too heavily on differential diagnoses and treatment options as we feel this is best covered by local or national guidelines that are frequently updated.

This guide is designed for you to dip in and out of as questions arise during daily clinical practice. Much of the text is written in bullet point form with key words highlighted in bold to allow you to quickly find the information you need. Throughout the book the 'Top Tips' boxes provide helpful practical suggestions and highlight common pitfalls to avoid. Also, words that READ LIKE THIS are defined in the jargon buster section of Chapter 1.

We wrote this book for all doctors who see children as their patients, not just those working in paediatrics. Those working in general practice, the emergency department and some surgical specialties such as orthopaedics and ENT are particularly likely to find this book of great help when seeing their younger patients. We have also included a chapter called 'Developing Your Career' to provide advice about how to pass exams, outlining the structure of paediatric training and how to get ahead for junior doctors and medical students considering a career in paediatrics.

With one of us a junior doctor and the other an experienced consultant paediatrician and educator, we have been able to write from two perspectives: knowing how it feels 'not to know' and writing 'all the things I wish I'd known' and combining this with the insight gained from many years of clinical practice and teaching. We hope that you will enjoy using this book and that it will help you to develop the skills and knowledge to provide the best possible care for children and their families.

Rebecca Hewitson
Caroline Fertleman

Acknowledgements

The authors would like to thank the following people for their help and advice:

Lee Anthony, Nirit Braha, Juan Carrasco-Alvarez, Jo Carroll, Rahul Chodhari, Michael Clift, Zayne Crow, Rebecca Crowe, Sarah Eisen, Ian Evans, Anthony Gaerets, Benjamin Harold, Katerina Harris, Jayne Kavanagh, Chris Knapp, Silvana Kohon, Chloe Macaulay, Mark Madams, Maxine Phelops, Sunita Rao and Eleanor Tickner.

The following figures and excerpts have been reproduced with permission from the publishers:

Department of Education, HM Government (2013) *Working Together to Safeguard Children* (under Crown copyright licence)
Figures 4.1, 4.2, 4.3 and 4.4

Resuscitation Council UK (2010) *Resuscitation Guidelines*.
Figures 5.1, 5.6, 5.10 and 9.1

Advanced Life Support Group (2011) *Advanced Paediatric Life Support*, 5th edn. Wiley-Blackwell, Oxford.
Figures 5.14 and 5.16

About the companion website

Check out the

Hands-on Guide
to Practical Paediatrics
companion website at:

www.wileyhandsonguides.com/paediatrics

Click now to access:

- ■ practice prescribing scenarios with model answers and printable drug chart
- ■ videos demonstrating practical procedures
- ■ downloadable illustrations from the book
- ■ useful information in printable format to attach to your ID badge such as:
- – normal observations values
- – immunisation schedule
- – commonly used drug doses
- – Advanced Life Support formulas.

Chapter 1
GETTING STARTED

Who's who?

There are many different people on the children's ward, some of whom have jobs unique to dealing with children. This can be a little daunting at first if you're not sure what they all do and means that you have a lot of names to learn. However, having such a large and varied team means that collectively, you can provide much better care for your patients and their families and you can learn a lot from your colleagues' expertise. Understanding a little bit about what everyone in the team does will allow you to make the best use of their skills. The list below gives a brief description of some of the roles within the team. They are listed in alphabetical order for ease of reference.

Breastfeeding advisor

Many breastfeeding supporters are mothers who have trained to provide breastfeeding advice on a voluntary basis. They have a wealth of knowledge and tips and are able to provide support to mothers who are having difficulty establishing breastfeeding.

Child protection nurse ✓

By law, each hospital or community trust must have a named nurse and a named doctor who are responsible for child protection. Child protection nurses are extremely knowledgeable and are a very useful first port of call for advice if you have any concerns about a child's welfare. They attend child protection and psychosocial meetings and will often provide training on child protection to other members of staff.

Clinical support worker

Sometimes also known as therapy helper or therapy assistant. Their role is to work alongside, and under the supervision of, allied health professionals (such as physiotherapists and occupational therapists) and help with therapy sessions by preparing equipment, getting the patient ready before the session and providing an extra pair of hands during therapy sessions.

Dietitian

The dietition can give advice on feeding and nutrition, including advising about parenteral nutrition regimes or dietary supplements. They are crucial in the

The Hands-on Guide to Practical Paediatrics, First Edition. Rebecca Hewitson and Caroline Fertleman.
© 2014 John Wiley & Sons, Ltd. Published 2014 by John Wiley & Sons, Ltd.
Companion Website: www.wileyhandsonguides.com/paediatrics

management of patients with eating disorders and can advise on monitoring for refeeding syndrome. They can also provide advice to children with food allergies.

Health visitor

Health visitors work in the community but you may come across them in the hospital at psychosocial meetings or when you are working in community paediatrics. Their work is varied but mostly involves going to visit families in their own homes. Health visitors routinely visit all new parents to provide any necessary advice or support in caring for their new baby. During these first few visits, they assess the level of support the parents need and decide how much longer they need to continue working with that family or if they need to refer on to other specialist services. They also play a vital role in supporting vulnerable children and families and are trained in recognising signs of abuse and neglect in children. They may be the first to raise concerns about the welfare of a child due to the valuable insight they gain from visiting families in their own homes.

Healthcare assistant

This is often abbreviated to HCA and HCAs are sometimes also known as auxiliary nurses or nurse auxiliaries. Their role is to work alongside nurses and midwives to provide them with support in their work. They will always be working under the supervision of a registered nurse or midwife. Duties involve things like helping with washing and dressing, meals, making beds and taking observations. The experience of healthcare assistants can vary a lot. Some may be working as a HCA whilst studying to become a registered nurse whilst others may have little or no medical knowledge. It is important to understand that the role and training level of healthcare assistants differ significantly from those of nurses (they are unable to dispense medications, for example).

Midwife

Midwifes have a varied role as they are involved in the care of pregnant women antenatally, the safety of mother and baby during labour and delivery, and the care of mother and baby in the early postnatal period. They are able to offer advice to mothers about feeding, supported by the breastfeeding advisor for women who need additional support. Some midwives are also trained to perform newborn baby checks.

Nursery assistant

Nursery assistants need no specific childcare qualifications but will assist nursery nurses in their work and under supervision. They can still provide very useful support to children by engaging them in play and distracting them from procedures but will not be able to help with more specialist work such as explaining diagnoses through play in the same way as a play specialist or nursery nurse would be able to.

Nursery nurse

Nursery nurses have many similar roles to the hospital play specialists but will often also work in community settings. In order to be a nursery nurse, they will have a childcare qualification but will not have trained to as high a level as a play specialist (who undergoes additional training). They may work alongside play specialists.

Occupational therapist

The role of the occupational therapist (also called an OT) is to help children to be able to do all the things that any child of their age could do. Essentially, their role involves assessing any physical or psychiatric IMPAIRMENT that the child may have and providing practical solutions to minimise the extent to which this impairment becomes a DISABILITY. This might mean making adaptations to the child's home or providing them with equipment or tools to help them to complete tasks.

Orthoptist

Orthoptists work within the ophthalmology team to help diagnose, investigate and treat problems with eye movements, such as squints (strabismus). Some are also involved in vision screening for children in community health centres and schools.

Pharmacist

The ward pharmacist is an enormously useful source of information so make good use of them. They will be able to advise you on the latest research on certain medications, the most effective preparations to use and possible side-effects to be aware of, and can help you with difficult prescriptions. They also check all the drug charts and may spot mistakes you have made in your prescriptions. Try not to take this as a criticism but instead be grateful that they have pointed it out to you so that you have the chance to correct it and try to learn from their advice. They are also very useful for communicating with families and GPs to establish exactly which regular medications a child takes and to discuss changes to medications with parents.

Pharmacy technician

Pharmacy technicians work closely with pharmacists to assemble, label and dispense medications. They check the stock of medications on the ward and expiry dates of medications. They are sometimes also involved in checking and recording the medications patients are taking and talking with families about how to use their medicines safely at home. They may not have the same depth of knowledge as pharmacists for helping with queries about prescriptions.

Physician assistant

Only present in a handful of paediatric centres but an incredibly valuable resource (count yourself very lucky if you have them at your hospital). They are trained to support doctors in the medical management of patients and can often perform blood tests and insert cannulas, check blood results, write discharge summaries and order investigations. As they take on some similar roles to junior doctors (but tend to be in the same post for longer), they become experts on the ins and outs of how the hospital works and can be vital to the smooth running of the department. There will be individual variation between what they are trained and comfortable doing so avoid making assumptions and ask.

Physiotherapist

Physiotherapists are highly trained and probably have a much better knowledge of working anatomy than you do. Physiotherapists help children with balance and mobility problems through exercises, manual therapy and provision of mobility aids (such as frames or wheelchairs). They can help with postural problems for children with spinal deformity, prevent joint contractures and also provide chest physiotherapy (for example, to help children with pneumonia to clear mucus from their airways).

Play specialist

Play specialists are experts in child development and age-appropriate play and will have had to study for several different qualifications (including a degree) in order to work as a hospital play specialist. They are crucial in helping to distract children whilst you are performing procedures and can help with the explanation of diagnoses and

treatments to children through engaging them in play. They can also provide support to siblings and contribute to clinical decisions based on the child's behaviour that they have observed whilst playing.

Psychologist

Child psychologists may specialise in either clinical or educational psychology. A clinical psychologist will be involved in the management of children with mental health problems such as anxiety and depression, those struggling to adjust to their physical illness or children with behavioural problems or issues with family relationships. Educational psychologists are more likely to work in a community setting. They aim to enhance the child's learning ability through helping them with their emotional problems or learning difficulties and have an important role in advising teachers, parents and social workers.

School teacher

Many children's departments will have a hospital school with a qualified teacher so that children do not fall behind with their education whilst they are inpatients. Teachers at hospital schools can be very helpful as part of the multidisciplinary team in identifying any ongoing special educational needs that the child may have. Some hospital schools have status as 'special schools' and teach children who are not currently inpatients but are not able to attend their normal school for medical reasons.

Specialist nurse

These are nurses who have specialised in a particular disease area and work solely with children and families with those diagnoses (for example, diabetes, cancer or sickle cell specialist nurses). They are incredibly knowledgeable in their area of expertise and are often involved in providing training to other healthcare staff, including doctors, on their specialist subject. They work closely with patients and families and can provide great continuity of care as they get to know their patients very well. Make sure that you inform them if a patient who is known to them is admitted so that they can come to review and offer advice. They are also enormously helpful in providing support to families whose child has been given a new diagnosis. Some specialist nurses may be independent practitioners who can manage children independently and prescribe medications.

Social worker

They provide support to vulnerable children and families in the community and also assess if a child is at risk of suffering abuse or neglect. They work closely with the multidisciplinary team in providing advice about children and families they are working with and attend regular psychosocial meetings at the hospital and in community settings as well as case conferences and child protection meetings. Good communication between social workers and hospital teams is crucial for managing child protection cases well. If you have concerns about the welfare of a child you can call the Child and Family social care team to ask for advice or make a formal referral. For more details see Chapter 4, Child Protection and Safeguarding. Social workers also have an important role in supporting children who have mental health problems such as those who are self-harming.

Speech and language therapist

Although speech and language therapists do have an important role to play in helping children who have difficulties developing speech (making the noise) and language (knowing the words), they do much more than this. They help children more broadly with communication, using communication aids such as symbol boards and voice synthesisers in order to help children who are having difficulties communicating. They are also crucial in helping with feeding issues, which isn't totally obvious from their job title but makes sense when you think about it. They are experts on all things to do with the physical process of producing speech – mouth, tongue, larynx, etc. – and so, given that they already know so much about this, the natural extension is for them to be involved with things like swallowing which involves much of the same anatomy.

Staff nurse

New nurses who are studying now are all trained to degree level and paediatric nurses tend to be particularly motivated and skilled individuals. Getting on well with the nursing staff is vital if you are going to provide good care for your patients as you will work more closely with them on a day-to-day basis than any other members of the multidisciplinary team.

Ward clerk

Ward clerks are responsible for requesting patient records and making sure that they are returned for storage after they have been used. They will file notes and chase up reports as well as answering phone calls and welcoming patients and families at a reception desk to the ward. They are likely to be able to book follow-up appointments for your patients, which can be really helpful for families to know as they leave rather than waiting for a letter. They can also track down missing notes for you and order stationery (such as replacement paper for the printer).

Ward sister

Ward sisters are senior and experienced paediatric nurses who are in charge of the day-to-day running of the ward. They supervise the nurses and healthcare assistants on the ward in addition to having lots of paperwork to complete and fulfilling their normal nursing duties. They are very busy people and their job can be extremely stressful so try to be considerate and not bother them unnecessarily when they are in the middle of something and don't take it personally if they are sometimes a little short with you when you do. They can be a great source of

advice and support when you are learning so don't be afraid to ask for their help.

What happens where?

As well as there being lots of different people on the ward there are also some rooms and special wards which are unique to paediatrics.

Playroom

Many paediatric wards will have a playroom and if you can't find one of your patients, this is usually the best place to start looking. It is really important for children to have time to play and many hospitals will have well-equipped playrooms with activities organised by play specialists.

Teenage room

Teenagers are unlikely to want to sit in the play room with lots of young, excited children. Many wards offer separate rooms for teenagers with more age-appropriate video games and reading material.

Treatment room

Unlike for adults, for whom most procedures are done at the bedside, this is avoided if possible for children. Procedures are not done at the bedside for young children unless absolutely necessary because it is important that they feel that their bed is a safe place. Children's wards will therefore have treatment rooms where children are taken to have procedures done. They are often decorated to try to make them as welcoming as possible.

School room

It is important that children continue to learn whilst they are in hospital so that they don't fall behind with their education and also to normalise the hospital experience as much as possible. For this reason, children's departments may have dedicated school rooms with a qualified teacher to provide lessons for inpatients.

Parents' room

Parents are encouraged to stay with their children whilst they are in hospital to make the whole experience less frightening (for both child and parent). Wards will often have a room for parents to sit, sometimes with basic facilities such as a kettle or a microwave.

Sensory room

Some wards will have a sensory room, with interesting lights and colours and soft padding on the floors. These are great for young children and those with learning difficulties to enjoy with their parents.

Day care unit

Most paediatric units will have a day care ward for children who only need to come in for treatment during the day time (for example, for antibiotics, a minor procedure or sedation and imaging) but can go home overnight. You may be asked to review children on the day unit or prescribe medications for them as part of your ward or on-call duties. Day units are sometimes also known as 'ambulatory units'.

Milk room

Neonatal wards usually have a dedicated room for preparation and storage of milk. This can be making up formula feeds or thawing out frozen breastmilk for feeding the babies on the ward.

Postnatal ward

This is where mothers and babies who are well will go after delivery. You may be asked to review babies on the postnatal ward if midwives have concerns and this is where you usually go to perform newborn baby checks prior to discharge.

Paediatric emergency department

Many hospitals will have a separate area for children coming to the emergency department and separate paediatric resuscitation rooms. Make sure that you know how to access the paediatric emergency department at your hospital and whether paediatric resuscitations take place in a dedicated children's area or in the main emergency department resuscitation area so that you know where to run to in the event of a crash call.

Be prepared

It can be useful to have some extra things with you when you're on the paediatric ward or on call.

■ **A small toy**. This just needs to be something colourful which will entertain a small child for a couple of minutes whilst you try to examine them. It doesn't have to be anything big or flashy. Lots of people will attach a small keyring to their stethoscope in the shape of an animal. Often this can double up as something else useful (for example, getting a toy which lights up with a bright white light for looking in throats, or is a clock with a second hand). If you actually hand the toy to the child for them to hold (rather than just look at) then make sure to clean it thoroughly afterwards for infection control reasons.

■ **Calculator**. Most people will have a calculator function on their phone but it is not always convenient to take your phone around with you on the ward. You may wish to invest in a miniature calculator to carry around with you.

■ **Stethoscope**. Obviously you need one of these. It's not necessary to get a paediatric stethoscope initially, adult ones will work just fine.

■ **Pen torch**. For looking more closely at rashes, checking pupillary reactions, looking in the back of throats or entertaining small children (lighting up the torch and then pretending to blow it out and letting go of the button so it turns off is a great way of engaging young children who will really want to have a go themselves).

■ **Watch with a second hand**. The problem with the bare below the elbow policy is that if you're not wearing a watch, you can't count respiratory and pulse rates. These are crucial parts of your assessment of any child so invest in either a fob watch with a second hand or a keyring with a watch on it that you can attach to your stethoscope.

Jargon Buster

Key: Each term that LOOKS LIKE THIS is a jargon buster!

32 PLUS 3 This is just an example of the actual numbers used but when people talk about a baby who was born at '32 plus 3', what they mean is that the baby was 32 (completed) weeks and 3 days gestation when he or she was born. This is often written as '32^{+3}' when it is recorded in the notes.

5 IN 1 Single vaccine against five different diseases: diphtheria, tetanus, pertussis, polio and *Haemophilus influenzae* type b.

ACHIEVING BEST EVIDENCE This is the guidance set out for police officers about the best way of interviewing children about crimes that they have been victim of or witness to. It is about asking open, non-leading questions in order to gain the most reliable story from the child. This is important in cases of abuse when taking a history too as you want to avoid asking any leading questions in your history taking. If you have asked the child leading questions, it may mean that their statements will be judged as less reliable by the courts and could alter the outcome of a court case.

ADLS This stands for activities of daily living. It refers to all the things that we all do every day like washing, eating, dressing and going to the toilet.

ALTE This stands for apparently life-threatening event and is the term used to refer to reported episodes (usually in young babies) of the child becoming floppy, blue and unresponsive.

BLOOD GAS Do not assume when people talk about blood gases in paediatrics that they are referring to an arterial blood gas. These are rarely done in children and a venous or capillary blood gas is much more likely to be used instead. *See Chapter 6 – Practical Procedures, for information on how to take a capillary blood gas sample.*

BODY MAP A standard blank diagram of a child's body on which you can draw any injuries or marks you have seen in the appropriate places. This makes it much easier to be accurate than trying to draw the child yourself or just using words to describe the size and location of marks. There are different body maps available for infants, older children and genitalia.

BURST THERAPY Giving three lots of salbutamol nebulisers and one lot of ipratropium nebulisers back to back to a child presenting with asthma.

CAIT If you hear people referring to 'CAIT' they may not be talking about a person called Kate, but about the Child Abuse Investigation Team! This is a specialised team of police officers who investigate possible criminal offences related to the abuse of children.

CAF You may hear people talking about 'caf' forms. This stands for 'Common Assessment Framework'. These are often used for communicating child protection concerns to social services in writing (usually following a phone conversation with them about the case).

CAFCASS This stands for Child and Family Court Advisory and Support Service. This is an organisation which provides support and advice to families going through court proceedings. Their social workers act as advocates for children and help to advise the courts as to what is in that child's best interests. Their website (www.cafcass.gov.uk) has lots of information written specifically for children, teenagers and families about the support that CAFCASS provides and the processes involved in court proceedings.

CAMHS You may hear people referring to 'cams'. This stands for 'Child and Adolescent Mental Health Services'.

CAPILLARY REFILL TIME This is often abbreviated to CRT. It is a way of assessing any problems with the child's circulation by looking at skin perfusion. It is best measured centrally (usually over the sternum) as the peripheral measurement can vary depending on the room temperature. Press down for 5 sec and then remove your finger and count how long it takes for the skin to return to a normal colour. Anything less than 2 sec is normal.

CENTILES The lines on growth charts which document the range of normal growth for children. If a child's height is on the 98th centile, this means that only 2% of children this age will be taller.

CHAIN OF EVIDENCE If you take a sample, the result of which may end up being used as evidence in court, you must use the chain of evidence process for that sample. For example, if you suspect a sexually transmitted infection in a young child, the result of any swabs you take may subsequently be used to convict someone of sexual abuse. This means that it must be clear that this is the right result for the right patient. *For more about the chain of evidence process, see Chapter 4 under the Sexual abuse subheading.*

CHILD IN NEED A child in need is any child who will need input from services in order to reach or maintain a good standard of health and development. This means that all children with disabilities and LOOKED-AFTER CHILDREN are automatically defined as children in need. A child who is at significant risk of abuse or neglect is also a child in need. *For more about the child protection process, see Chapter 4 under Working with social services, education and the police.*

CHILD PROTECTION CONFERENCE This is a formal meeting that forms part of the assessment process if there are concerns that a child is subject to abuse or neglect. The meeting involves family members (including the child if appropriate), with any relevant supporters, advocates or professionals who have been involved with the child or the family. The purpose of the meeting is to decide if the child is at risk of significant harm in the future and therefore should be subject to a CHILD PROTECTION PLAN. *For more about the child protection process, see Chapter 4 under Working with social services, education and the police.*

CHILD PROTECTION PLAN This is a plan put in place for children who have been abused or neglected and who are at ongoing risk of harm. The plan outlines what needs to be done and by whom in order to keep the child safe. The type of abuse to which the child was being subjected is recorded as part of the plan (i.e. physical, sexual, etc.) and a lead social worker will be allocated to be in charge of the case and ensure that all the plans are implemented. *For more about the child protection process, see Chapter 4 under Working with social services, education and the police.*

CHILD PROTECTION REGISTER The child protection register used to be a list kept by the local authority of all children who were felt to be at risk of significant abuse but these lists no longer exist. You may well still hear people referring to a child being 'on the register' but this is outdated terminology. What they probably mean is that the child is 'subject to a CHILD PROTECTION PLAN'.

COMPENSATED SHOCK This expression tends to be used much more frequently in paediatrics than in adult medicine. Children have a greater physiological reserve than adults and so can compensate for shock very well for some time before rapidly deteriorating. Compensated shock means that the child is still managing to maintain perfusion of their vital organs but you need to intervene soon in order to prevent progression to DECOMPENSATED SHOCK. *For more about shock and resuscitation of acutely unwell children, see Chapter 5 – Common Paediatric Emergencies.*

CORE ASSESSMENT Sometimes also known as a section 47 enquiry, this is a detailed assessment led by social services in cases when a child is thought to be at risk of abuse or neglect. Social services work with police, health and education to gather information and conduct interviews with parents and the child. Health professionals may be asked to carry out detailed assessments of the child's development. The social worker then makes a decision about whether or not to convene a CHILD PROTECTION CONFERENCE. *For more about the child protection process, see Chapter 4 under Working with social services, education and the police.*

CORRECTED GESTATIONAL AGE (ABBREVIATED TO CGA) Also sometimes known as 'corrected uterine age', this is used for babies who are born prematurely. To work it out, add the number of days old the child is to the gestation they were when they were born, e.g. a baby born at 32^{+3} (i.e. 32 weeks and 3 days) who is now 13 days old would have a CGA of 34^{+2}. This is useful because how a baby behaves and likely medical issues and appropriate treatment will vary based on their gestational age rather than how long they have been out of the womb for, i.e. a 13-day-old TERM BABY will be vastly different from a 13-day -old baby born at 26 weeks' gestation in terms of size, physiology and development.

CRASH TROLLEY This is a portable trolley that contains all the equipment needed to resuscitate a patient. It usually has separate drawers for airway, breathing and circulation with all the necessary equipment for each of these, any emergency drugs that may be needed and a defibrillator. Find out where the crash trolley is in your workplace so that you know where to find it in a hurry. You should also be aware that there are usually separate crash trolleys for children with appropriately sized equipment and drug doses.

DECEREBRATE POSTURING This indicates brainstem damage and may signal that a respiratory arrest is imminent. It is a rigid posture with the arms and legs both extended and internally rotated, the neck extended and the back arched. If this posturing was preceded by DECORTICATE POSTURING, then it may indicate brain herniation (or 'coning') as a result of raised intracranial pressure. *See Chapter 5 – Common Paediatric Emergencies and Fig. 5.15 for more details.*

DECOMPENSATED SHOCK This is when a child is no longer able to maintain a sufficient blood pressure to perfuse their vital organs. Signs include hypotension, reduced consciousness and bradycardia. Decompensated shock is a life-threatening emergency and you should either put out a paediatric crash call or call the emergency services (2222 in hospital or 999 in the community). If a child has bradycardia, start Basic Life Support. *See Chapter 5 – Common Paediatric Emergencies for details.*

DECORTICATE POSTURING This indicates damage to the higher functioning portions of the brain such as the cere-bral cortex. It is a rigid posture in which the arms are flexed and the hands clenched in fists and the legs are extended and internally rotated. *See Chapter 5 – Common Paediatric Emergencies and Fig. 5.15 for more details.*

DEVELOPMENTAL DELAY This is when a child is much slower than expected for their age in acquiring certain skills. This can be specific to one particular area of development (for example, isolated delayed speech development) or a child can have 'global developmental delay', meaning that they are slow to develop in many different areas. *For more on child development see Chapter 2 – Child Development.*

DISABILITY A limitation of what a child is able to do relative to other healthy children of their age, as a result of an impairment. The environment in which a child lives affects the extent to which their IMPAIRMENT becomes a disability. For example, a child who is a triple amputee may have excellent prostheses and not be limited at all in their activities (it is even possible to snowboard with prosthetic limbs) but a child with poor vision who does not have access to glasses could be very disabled because of this impairment. In developed countries, most poor vision is not considered a disability at all because use of glasses to correct it is widespread, but these individuals would have limited function without them.

DYSMORPHIC The term used to describe babies who have unusual facial features. Dysmorphic features tend to occur as a group of unusual characteristics together as part of a genetic syndrome (such as flattened nasal bridge and a protruding tongue in children with Down syndrome).

EMERGENCY PROTECTION ORDER (EPO) These can be applied for urgently from the court in cases where there is concern that a child is in immediate danger. If the Emergency Protection Order is granted by the courts, it gives the local authority the right to remove the child from their home to a place of safety. The EPO lasts for 8 days, during which time the local authority has parental responsibility for the child and can give consent to medical treatment on the child's behalf if necessary.

EX-PREM A baby or child who was born prematurely but now has a corrected gestation equivalent to a **TERM BABY** or older.

FAILURE TO THRIVE This is when a baby or child does not gain weight or grow at the rate they would be expected to. This can mean slow weight gain, no weight gain or even weight loss. There are many diagnoses that can be responsible for failure to thrive or it may simply be a result of the child not receiving adequate nutrition.

FEMALE GENITAL MUTILATION (COMMONLY ABBREVIATED TO FGM) A general term referring to any process involving removal or injury of the external female genitalia for non-medical reasons. It can involve anything from cutting or piercing the genital area to total removal of the clitoris and labia minora or surgical narrowing of the vaginal opening. It may be referred to by families as 'cutting' or 'female circumcision'.

FRASER GUIDELINES A set of guidelines laid out by Lord Fraser to help doctors make decisions about when a child under 16 years old may be capable of giving consent for contraception or an abortion.

GILLICK COMPETENCE The term used to refer to children under the age of 16 who are thought to be capable of consenting to treatment themselves (without the need for parental consent). In order for a child to be deemed 'Gillick Competent', they must be able to understand the facts about the treatment, understand the consequences of the treatment or of not having the treatment and be able to weigh up these factors in order to come to a reasoned decision. The name 'Gillick Competence' arose following a case of a mother, Victoria Gillick, who went to the courts to seek a ruling that doctors could not prescribe contraception for her daughters who were under 16 without her consent. The House of Lords ruled against Gillick and determined that a parent was not able to overrule medical decisions made by a young person if they were able to fully understand the treatment that was proposed and therefore give consent themselves.

GLOBAL DEVELOPMENTAL DELAY See 'developmental delay' above.

GRID TRAINING You might hear people talking about how they are applying for 'the grid' or 'grid training'. This basically means that they are applying to train in a subspecialty of paediatrics. *For more information about grid training, see Chapter 11 – Developing Your Career.*

GUEDEL AIRWAY Also known as an oropharyngeal airway, this is a curved plastic tube which can be used to keep a child's airway open if the child has reduced conscious level.

HEEL PRICK This is a way of taking blood from babies and toddlers by using a lancet to form a small cut in the skin, allowing you to collect drops of blood by squeezing and encouraging the cut to bleed. This is usually done on the fleshy part of the heel (hence the name). *For more about blood sampling, see Chapter 6 – Practical Procedures.*

IMPAIRMENT A physical, cognitive or sensory abnormality.

INITIAL ASSESSMENT This is also known as a section 17 investigation. When a social worker receives a referral from someone who is worried about the child's welfare, they may decide that further investigation of the concern is needed. This is called an initial assessment. They will contact multiple different agencies (education, police, etc.) to gather information about the child's social circumstances and may also contact the person who made the referral to find out more detail about their concerns. They will also conduct interviews with the child and their family. After they have completed their assessment, they will make a decision about whether or not that child is a CHILD IN NEED.

ISAM You might hear people referring to an 'eye-sam' baby. This is an abbreviation for infant of substance-abusing mother and refers to babies with neonatal abstinence syndrome (see Chapter 4). This is a terrible abbreviation so try to avoid using it yourself.

JABS An informal word used for immunisations.

LOOKED-AFTER CHILD A looked-after child is one for whom the local authority is responsible. This normally means that the local authority shares PARENTAL RESPONSIBILITY with the child's parents and that the local authority are responsible for finding a suitable place for the child to live (usually, with suitable relative, in a care home or with a foster family).

MAINTENANCE PLUS 5% This refers to a child who is 5% dehydrated and needs IV fluid replacement above the normal maintenance amount. It is calculated using a special formula; *see the section on replacement therapy in Chapter 7 for details.* It does *not* mean that you simply calculate their maintenance fluid volume and then add an additional 5% to that volume – this is incorrect and a common mistake!

MEMBERSHIP OR MRCPCH These both refer to the same thing which is the process of passing several exams in order to be allowed to practise as a registrar in paediatrics. Successfully passing all the exams gains you membership of the Royal College of Paediatrics and Child Health or MRCPCH for short. This is the qualification to say that you can practise as a paediatrician.

MICROTAINERS These are paediatric blood bottles which are much smaller than adult bottles and only need 1 mL of blood to fill them.

NEONATE A neonate is a baby who is less than 1 month old.

NICU Often pronounced 'nickoo', this stands for neonatal intensive care unit.

NIPE You may hear people talking about 'ny-pea' – they are referring to the Newborn and Infant Physical Examination Programme (NIPE) which includes software used to record the outcome of newborn baby checks.

NPA This stands for nasopharyngeal aspirate, a procedure that involves suctioning secretions from a baby's or child's nose into a specimen pot that is sent to the laboratory for analysis. Nasopharyngeal aspirates are used to determine the causative organism of a respiratory infection (most commonly respiratory syncytial virus).

OOPE When people are talking about an 'oo-pee', they are probably referring to an Out of Programme Experience. This is an opportunity to take time out of the paediatric programme to pursue other interests (such as research or working abroad) or for personal reasons (such as childcare or ill health).

PARENTAL RESPONSIBILITY This is a legal definition referring to someone who is responsible for making important decisions about a child's life such as where they go to school, where they live and whether or not to undergo medical treatments. Married couples both automatically have parental responsibility and this remains even if the couple divorce. Unmarried mothers automatically have parental responsibility but unmarried fathers do not. Others, such as stepparents, adoptive parents or the local authority, can acquire parental responsibility following application through the courts. *For more details about parental responsibility and consent, see Chapter 3 – Communication with Children and their Parents.*

PEWS Often pronounced in the same way as a church bench rather than the letters spelled out. PEWS stands for Paediatric Early Warning Score. It is a way of efficiently communicating between members of the team how well or unwell a child is based on their observations. A PEWS score for a normal, healthy child is 0 (i.e. all their observations are within normal range). The higher the PEWS score, the more unwell the child. The maximum score is 6.

PICU Sometimes said as the individual letters, sometimes pronounced 'pickoo'. This stands for paediatric intensive care unit.

PREDUCTAL SATURATIONS This refers to measuring the oxygen saturation levels in the right hand of newborn babies. This is because this reflects the 'preductal' circulation, i.e. the blood pumped from the left side of the heart, before it mixes with blood from the right side via the ductus arteriosus, which remains patent for a short time after birth. For this reason you would expect the oxygen saturation levels to be slightly higher if measured in the right hand rather than the left hand or the feet, as the brachiocephalic artery (which supplies the right arm) branches from the aorta before the ductus arteriosus.

QIP People sometimes pronounce this 'quip'. It stands for quality improvement project which is what it sounds like – a project to try to improve the quality of some aspect of care provided to patients or the efficiency with which the hospital runs. These can be very effectively lead by junior doctors. They are a bit like audits, but for cases where you're not comparing practice to a known standard but coming up with a new solution to a problem. This can be much more exciting than completing an audit by giving you a chance to be innovative and have an impact on patient care.

RED BOOK Also known as a personal child health record. All parents are given a red book with their newborn baby. This is a parent-held health record for that child which contains growth charts, details of immunisations and developmental milestones, amongst other things. It can be filled in by healthcare professionals and parents.

REGRESSION If a child is described as 'regressing' this means that they have lost the ability to do things that they could previously do. This is very worrying as it can reflect a serious underlying neurodegenerative condition. It is normal for children to behave slightly younger than they normally would when they are unwell or frightened or following the birth of a new sibling but regression refers to a permanent loss of skills, not just a temporary change in behaviour.

RESUSCITAIRE Resuscitaires are the mini workstations/platforms with all the gadgetry you may need for resuscitating a newborn attached to them.

SBAR Often pronounced 'ess-bar', this is a structure to aid communication between team members. It stands for Situation, Background, Assessment and Recommendations. *For more information about using SBAR, see Chapter 10 – Looking After Yourself.*

SBR Stands for spun bilirubin, a quick way of getting a result for total bilirubin levels in a serum sample. Usually performed using machines on the ward by clinical staff (*see Chapter 6 – Practical Procedures*). If you send a sample to the laboratory you will get a breakdown of the conjugated and unconjugated fraction of bilirubin too.

SCBU Sometimes pronounced 'skuh-boo', this stands for special care baby unit. It is for neonates who still need to be in hospital but do not require as much intensive or specialist treatment as babies on the intensive care unit.

SECTION 17 INVESTIGATION See 'initial assessment'.

SECTION 47 INVESTIGATION See 'core assessment'.

SEE-SAW BREATHING This is when a child is attempting to breathe against an obstructed or partially obstructed airway. This results in their abdomen moving out and their chest wall moving in as they attempt to breathe in. It is a worrying sign as it suggests airway obstruction.

SPA This stands for suprapubic aspirate. This is a method of collecting a urine sample by using a needle to enter the bladder through the anterior abdominal wall. *For more about how to do this procedure, see Chapter 6 – Practical Procedures.*

STATEMENT OF SPECIAL EDUCATIONAL NEEDS This is a document put together for a child with complex or severe difficulties following assessment by the local education authority. It details what the child's educational needs are and what support they will need. It is reviewed annually.

STRATEGY DISCUSSION/STRATEGY MEETING This is the step after an **INITIAL ASSESSMENT** in the child protection process. It can be in the form of a meeting or can be done with separate phone calls to each of the agencies by the social worker. As a minimum, it must involve a social worker and their manager, a police officer and a health professional but may include other relevant people such as the person who made the referral and teachers from the child's school or nursery. This is used as a way of everyone sharing relevant information which allows decisions to be made about whether any immediate action is needed to keep the child safe,

whether a **CORE ASSESSMENT** should take place and if and when any criminal investigation will take place.

STRETCHING Stretching a child may sound like physiotherapy or a form of torture but in fact it relates to 'stretching' the time between nebulisers for children with asthma, e.g. 'stretching' from 2-hourly to 4-hourly nebulisers for a child whose wheeze seems to be improving.

SUPERVISED LEARNING EVENTS Sometimes abbreviated to SLE. This is just a different expression sometimes used for work-based assessments (see below).

TERM BABY Baby born at or after 37 weeks' gestation.

TERTIARY CENTRE You will probably be familiar with the terms primary and secondary care (referring to community-based and hospital-based care respectively). Tertiary care is the next level up. Tertiary centres provide super-specialist care which is not available at most hospitals. There are many fewer places which provide tertiary care, meaning that families sometimes have to travel quite long distances for these services.

WAFTING OXYGEN In situations when a young child has a partially obstructed airway it is really important not to upset them as this can result in total occlusion of their airway. Ideally, you want to give high-flow oxygen to children with airway compromise but you also want to avoid upsetting young children who do not like having a mask fitted. In this situation, the child shouldn't be forced to wear the mask but instead you can ask their parent to hold the mask near to the child's face in an attempt to slightly increase their inspired oxygen concentration. This is sometimes referred to as 'wafting oxygen'.

WORKPLACE-BASED ASSESSMENTS This is sometimes shortened to WBAs or WPBAs. These are not exams but formative assessments which you must complete on a regular basis at work in order to show how you are progressing. There are several different types of assessments but this is the umbrella term used for all of them. *For more about work-based assessments, see Chapter 11 – Developing Your Career.*

Chapter 2
CHILD DEVELOPMENT

If you haven't spent much time with children, it can be really difficult to know what, for example, your average one year old can do (or even how big you might expect them to be). Knowing roughly what to expect at what age will help you to get children to co-operate and avoid embarrassment in front of parents. For example, trying to distract a 2 year old by suggesting they count how many fish they can see in a picture can leave you red-faced when you realise they are unable to do this at that age. Knowing the subtleties of child development is a specialty in itself but having a grasp of the basics is crucial as if a child is not growing or developing normally, it can indicate an underlying problem.

Something vital to have in your mind when reviewing a child who you think may have **DEVELOPMENTAL DELAY** is 'could this be a symptom of abuse?'. A child who is ignored at home may be delayed in their development (particularly in speech and language). Also, you need to be able to spot when the story given by a parent doesn't fit with the child's age (a 4 week old could not have hurt themselves by 'rolling off the sofa' as they are unable to roll at this age).

Please see Chapter 4 – Child Protection and Safeguarding for more details on signs of child abuse.

There is some variation in the age at which children do certain things but the important thing is to know when you may need to refer for a specialist opinion. Below we'll go through different age groups, looking at what they can normally do and worrying signs which should prompt you to get a senior review.

What can a child of this age normally do?

Development is normally divided into four different areas of skills: gross motor, fine motor and vision, hearing and speech, and social. You may be asked to consider this when presenting information to other people if you think that there is a problem with one particular group of skills. *See Table 2.1 for when to worry that a child's development is delayed and possible underlying causes.*

The Hands-on Guide to Practical Paediatrics, First Edition. Rebecca Hewitson and Caroline Fertleman.
© 2014 John Wiley & Sons, Ltd. Published 2014 by John Wiley & Sons, Ltd.
Companion Website: www.wileyhandsonguides.com/paediatrics

Table 2.1 When to worry that a child's development is delayed.

Milestone	Limit age	Potential cause
Smile	10 weeks	Abnormal vision Neurological problem
Fix and follow	3 months	Abnormal vision
Reaching for objects Passing objects hand to hand	6 months 8 months	Abnormal vision Musculoskeletal problem Neurological problem
Sitting unsupported	12 months	Musculoskeletal problem Neurological problem
Pincer grip	12 months	Visual problem Co-ordination problem Gross motor problem
Walking unsupported	18 months	Musculoskeletal problem Neurological problem 'Bottom shuffler'
Uses spoon to self-feed	18 months	Co-ordination problem Musculoskeletal problem Neurological problem Lack of stimulus
Six words	18 months	Hearing problem Motor disorder Austistic spectrum disorder Lack of stimulus
'Handedness' – a preference for using one hand over the other	No *younger* than 18 months	Musculoskeletal problem or neurological problem affecting less used side
Symbolic play	2.5 years	Austistic spectrum disorder
Running	2.5 years	Co-ordination problem Musculoskeletal problem
Speech intelligible by strangers	3 years	Hearing problems Co-ordination problems

In order to be able to identify what is abnormal, you need to have an idea of what a normal child of that age can do. Below are descriptions of what children can normally do at certain ages.

Six weeks

By 6 weeks babies start to gain some control over their head movements and should be able to move their heads from side to side when lying on their fronts. Newborn babies have very blurry vision and cannot 'fix' on objects with their eyes but by 6 weeks their vision will have developed enough to allow them to 'fix and follow', i.e. focus on an object placed in the centre of their vision and turn their head to the left or right to follow the object with their gaze as it moves. Babies are particularly interested in faces and will be more likely to focus on a face than any other object.

From 6 weeks of age babies start to learn to smile. Don't expect to always be able to elicit this on examination – ask the parents if baby has been smiling in response to them.

Six to eight months

By 6 months most babies will be able to sit up. They may still be needing support to sit initially but by 8 months most will sit unsupported. They should be reaching out for and grabbing at objects with the palm of their hand and able to hold simple objects; they will also be developing the ability to transfer objects from hand to hand.

By this age babies should be making babbling noises and turning their head to noises out of sight. From 6 months, babies start learning how to feed themselves by picking up food with their hands and start to put everything they pick up in their mouths.

Twelve months

By the time babies reach one year old, they should be able to pull themselves to a standing position and start 'cruising' around the furniture (travelling around the room on their feet by grabbing onto furniture with their hands to help them balance). Some children will even be able to walk unsupported by this age (albeit rather unsteadily). They will use a pincer grip (between thumb and fingers) to pick up objects, will be able to wave bye-bye and play peek-a-boo. They will probably be able to say one or two words and understand their name.

Eighteen months

At 18 months old, children should be able to walk independently and may be able to start running a little too. They can hold a crayon to draw random scribbles and build a small tower of bricks (2–4 cubes). They may be starting to use one hand in preference to the other but if this has occurred any earlier than 18 months, this is a worrying sign as it may represent a problem with the side they are not using. They will be able to use between six and 12 words and will be able to use a spoon to feed themselves. At this age children also start to use 'symbolic play', e.g. pretending to cook.

Two years

By the time children are 2 years old they are much more steady on their feet and should be able to run around and may be able to kick a ball and jump. They will be able to say more words and will start joining two or three words together to express what they want, e.g. 'give me teddy'. Most will know five or six body parts, which can be helpful when trying to examine them ('where is your tummy?') and will be able to remove items of clothing. At this age they may start with potty training and be dry by day.

Three years

By 3 years of age children can handle three wheels – they will be able to ride a tricycle. Most children at this age can walk up and down stairs (but will probably still have to use two feet on each step on the way back down). Most can draw a circle and build a tower of nine bricks or a little bridge out of three blocks.

Many 3 year olds will chat almost constantly to their parents in three- or four-word sentences and ask a lot of questions. They are able to play with other children and start to understand the concept of taking turns. Most will be fairly independent with toileting, but they won't be able to wipe themselves effectively at this age.

It goes without saying that children continue to develop after the age of 3 but the obvious big milestones (in terms of motor and language skills) mostly happen within those first few years when skills develop very rapidly. After this it becomes a case of refining the skills that they have learnt.

School

School plays a crucial role in a child's development and is a big part of their life, so knowing which year group a child belongs to at which age can be helpful in discussions with children and parents. In the UK school starts and finishes at slightly different ages between the different countries, as does progression between 'primary' and 'secondary' education (in some areas children go to 'middle school' between primary and secondary). It may be worth finding out what is the case in your local area as education systems and rules can change. Table 2.2 provides a rough cheat sheet to give you an idea.

Developmental delay and children with disabilities

A child's development can be delayed in relation to one specific skill or across all developmental aspects (global delay).

Top Tip

Delay in acquiring certain skills is very different from a child losing the ability to do something which they could do previously. This is referred to as the child 'REGRESSING' and can indicate a serious neurodegenerative condition.

Table 2.2 Age ranges of primary and secondary school years in England and Wales, Scotland and Northern Ireland.

| | Year group at school | | |
Child's age	England and Wales	Scotland	Northern Ireland
Primary education			
4–5 years	Reception	Primary 1	P1
5–6 years	Year 1	Primary 2	P2
6–7 years	Year 2	Primary 3	P3
7–8 years	Year 3	Primary 4	P4
8–9 years	Year 4	Primary 5	P5
9–10 years	Year 5	Primary 6	P6
10–11 years	Year 6	Primary 7	P7
Secondary education			
11–12 years	Year 7	S1 (First year)	Year 8 (First year)
12–13 years	Year 8	S2 (Second year)	Year 9 (Second year)
13–14 years	Year 9	S3 (Third year)	Year 10 (Third year)
14–15 years	Year 10	S4 (Fourth year)	Year 11 (Fourth year)
15–16 years	Year 11	S5 (Fifth year)	Year 12 (Fifth year)
16–17 years	Year 12	S6 (Sixth year)	Year 13 (Lower sixth)
17–18 years	Year 13		

GLOBAL DEVELOPMENTAL DELAY usually becomes apparent within the first 2 years of a child's life. It is often associated with a degree of cognitive IMPAIRMENT but this may only become apparent in later years.

Many children with DEVELOPMENTAL DELAY will have an underlying medical condition and referral for detailed assessment early on is crucial. Diagnosis can allow treatment to start for the child and genetic counselling for parents if an inherited illness is diagnosed.

In 2007 the United Nations Children's Fund (UNICEF) published *Promoting the Rights of Children with Disabilities* (Innocenti Research Centre 2007). It opens with this paragraph:

'Children with disabilities and their families constantly experience barriers to the enjoyment of their basic human rights and to their inclusion in society. Their abilities are overlooked, their capacities are underestimated and their needs are given low priority. Yet, the barriers they face are more frequently as a result of the environment in which they live than as a result of their impairment.' (Reproduced by permission of UNICEF – Office of Research)

So how can you make sure that you don't become another barrier along the way? Here are some suggestions.

■ **Avoid making assumptions** about what a child is or is not able to do.

■ **Talk to the child too**. Just as you would with any other child, don't just ignore them and talk to the parents. Help them find ways to communicate with you if possible.

■ **They are the experts**. Parents of children with long-term conditions often become experts on their child's health problems and it is vital that they are treated as such. *For tips on how to communicate well with expert parents, see Chapter 3 – Communication with Children and Their Parents.*

■ **Be patient**. It is incredibly hard work looking after a child who is profoundly disabled, particularly for parents who have other children to look after as well. Be patient, even (and especially) if they are rude to you; they may be reaching the end of their tether. Contact a Family is a national UK charity with a great website to refer parents to if they don't know of it already (www.cafamily.org.uk). The charity has a freephone national helpline and a website with lots of information on medical conditions and can point parents towards where they can access support in their local area. It is also worth having a look yourself at the information for professionals available on the website.

■ **Be sensitive**. A child may have DEVELOPMENTAL DELAY as a result of an illness or injury and have been developing normally before that. Be sensitive when talking to parents about this – they may have had to repeat the story hundreds of times to different health professionals each time their child needs medical attention and it can be stressful and painful recalling what happened.

■ **Do your homework**. This child may be very well known to your hospital from multiple previous attendances. Rather than making parents go through all of it again, try having a look at a recent clinic or discharge letter which summarises the child's past medical history and ongoing medical problems. If you feel that you need to clarify with the parents, you could always show them a copy and ask if everything is up to date and if they want to add anything. Even if the child hasn't been seen at your hospital before, it is worth asking the parents if they have a summary of their child's illnesses and medications with them (many will have an organised and printed list with them detailing everything you need to know).

■ **Be alert**. Children with disabilities are much more prone to abuse – be alert to signs that their parents are not coping, for physical signs on examination of the child or for a change in the child's behaviour from their normal selves. *For more information, see Chapter 4 – Child Protection and Safeguarding.*

Support for children with disabilities and their families

Children with disabilities can have complex needs, both health and otherwise. This means that lots of different organisations are involved in supporting them (health, education, social services and voluntary services) and making sure that they communicate effectively with one another is difficult. This can be a source of enormous frustration for families when it doesn't work well.

Child development team

Child development services aim to have lots of different professionals under one roof to try to help communication between them and also to make services easier for families to access. A child development team normally consists of the following people: community paediatrician, speech and language therapist, occupational therapist, physiotherapist, psychologist, special needs teacher, health visitor and social worker. *For more information about what each of these people does as part of their job, see Chapter 1 – Getting Started.* The main aims of the child development team are to provide a diagnosis, medical management and refer for genetic counselling if appropriate. Many child development teams will only see children with complex needs who require access to more than one of their services.

Social services

All children with disabilities are considered to be 'CHILDREN IN NEED' and therefore must be assessed by social services in order to establish what extra support they may need. Social services must keep a register of children with disabilities and help to ensure that services for the child are well co-ordinated.

Education

Children with disabilities must be offered the opportunity to attend mainstream school and the school is legally obliged to make 'reasonable adjustments' in order to support the child in doing so if this is what the family wishes. This can vary from making physical adjustments to ensure that a child in a wheelchair can get to lessons to providing one-to-one support in the classroom and at break times.

Some families prefer their child to attend a special school where all the members of staff have expertise and class sizes are much smaller.

There is debate about whether mainstream schooling or special schools are better for children with disabilities. It is vital to listen to the wishes of the child and their parents when considering what will work best in each case.

If a child has complex or severe difficulties then the local education authority is legally obliged to perform an assessment for that child in order to establish what the child's educational needs are and what support they require. The authority will produce a document called a STATEMENT OF SPECIAL EDUCATIONAL NEEDS which is reviewed annually.

Finances

Caring for a child with disabilities is expensive for a whole host of different reasons. Parents may have reduced income from reducing hours or giving up work completely to look after the child and at the same time have increased costs of multiple trips to the hospital, specialist equipment and sometimes even needing to move to a bigger house in order to accommodate all the new equipment.

There are many different types of financial support available from the state to help cover some of these costs. Contact a Family has helpful information on its website about the different kinds of benefits available as does the UK government website (www.gov.uk) in its 'help if you have a disabled child' guide. The Family Fund (www.familyfund.org.uk) provides special grants for children with disabilities in the UK for one-off costs.

There are also many voluntary organisations who may be able to provide support by giving families specialist equipment or advice about what they are entitled to access from the state.

The Disabled Living Foundation's website (www.livingmadeeasy.org.uk/children) has information about what funding is available for buying children's equipment (from the state and the charity sector).

Transition

Transition to adult services is difficult and needs to be planned carefully. Transfer of information to adult services is crucial to avoid patients being investigated all over again for the same condition. People with learning difficulties are considered children until the age of 21 and once within adult services, there may well be a named learning disabilities specialist nurse who can offer support.

Growth

Keeping a record of how a child is growing is a crucial indicator for their underlying health. This means that measuring head circumference, length and weight (for babies) and weight and height (once over 2 years of age and able to stand) should be a routine part of any examination of a child and you should get into the habit of plotting these numbers on a growth chart.

It is important to know how to measure these things properly and also how to plot them on the growth charts. There are special growth charts available for children with certain conditions (such as Down and Turner syndrome) as they will be expected to grow at a different rate from other children. There are also charts available for Body Mass Index (more about this in the obesity section later in this chapter). See Box 2.1 for details of how to use growth charts properly.

Isolated measurements are less important than the trend of growth a child is showing. Children with normal growth should follow a centile line when you plot their growth (until they reach puberty when growth accelerates). For example, if a child has been following the 50th centile for weight

---

Box 2.1   How to measure and plot growth

Weight
- ■ Weigh babies naked (a wet nappy could change their weight significantly)
- ■ Weigh older children in only their underwear
- ■ Make sure that the scales you are using have been properly calibrated

Head circumference
- ■ Use a tape measure which is not stretchy! Most units have disposable paper versions
- ■ Measure around most prominent part of the occiput to the most prominent part of the forehead
- ■ Take the tape off and reposition to take three measurements
- ■ Record the largest of the three measurements as the head circumference

Length
- ■ If a child is less than 2 years old you should measure their length instead of their height.
- ■ You need a special piece of equipment and two people in order to do this properly
- ■ This can be really tricky to do well and often best to have an experienced person help you if length needs to be measured

Height
- ■ From 2 years onwards you can measure a child's height
- ■ Measure the child's height with no shoes on
- ■ Make sure that their knees and heels are flat against the wall or back of the measuring frame
- ■ Use a proper standing frame to measure the child's height
- ■ Lift slightly at the child's head to encourage them to stand straight but make sure they keep their feet flat on the floor

(Continued)

and then the latest value plots them on the 25th, you may not be initially concerned but plan to reweigh them in a few months' time. If their subsequent weight is below the 25th centile then this might be more of a cause for concern as the trend is continuing downwards. If a child's height or weight drops by two or more CENTILES then you certainly need to be discussing this with someone senior.

As well as looking at the trends, it is also important to consider the relationship between the different measurements. As a general rule, a child's measurements for height and weight should not be more than two CENTILES different from one another. Similarly, if a baby has a birth weight on the 50th centile but a head circumference on the second, this would warrant further investigation.

child's height all lie on, or very near, the 50th centile line then just say, for example, 'this child's height is following the 50th centile'. If, when you plot the dot on the graph, it lies between two centile lines then say so, e.g. 'between 50th and 75th CENTILES for height'. Don't try to estimate how far between those two lines they are and say 'they're on about the 65th centile' as the graphs cannot be interpreted in this way and people will wonder what you are talking about.

Obesity

Obesity in children is increasingly common; the UK and the Health Survey for England 2011 found that 31% of boys and 28% of girls aged 2–15 years were overweight or obese (Health and Social Care Information Centre 2013). There are many health implications for children who are overweight such as type 2 diabetes and hypertension, and their weight can also mean that they are subject to bullying and have low self-esteem.

Top Tip

You need to know how to talk about CENTILES when discussing a child's growth with other health professionals. If the dots for a

The National Institute for Health and Clinical Excellence (NICE) guidance in 2006 on tackling obesity in adults and children over 2 had recommendations for local authorities, schools and nurseries as well as health professionals (National Collaborating Centre for Primary Care and the Centre for Public Health Excellence 2006). According to this NICE guidance, children should be encouraged to do 60 min of moderate activity every day. This is quite a lot if a child is driven to and from school, chooses not to exercise during their school break times and then watches television when they get home from school. Limitations of safe outdoor space to play in (both in school and at home) can be one problem which needs to be overcome in achieving this.

 Top Tip

Children who are obese tend to be tall (because they are receiving more nourishment than needed for growth) but will also enter puberty earlier, meaning that their final height may not be that tall. If a child's centile for weight is much greater than their centile for height or their growth in height is faltering before reaching the final stages of puberty then consider a pathological cause for their obesity and work out their Body Mass Index (BMI).

The key to avoiding obesity in theory is simple: eat healthily and exercise more, but the social context and barriers which prevent this from happening are multiple and complex. This means that input is needed from lots of different places in order to tackle the problem, but health professionals have the privileged position of being trusted by patients and families and given authority to offer advice on health and can play an important part in raising the issue and pointing out where families can find help.

Given the statistics, you are very likely to meet some children who are overweight and obese, even if this is not their presenting problem. Knowing how best to start talking about it without being insensitive is difficult, but not acting can have much more devastating consequences for the child. It may not always be appropriate to discuss in the acute setting but don't use this as a regular excuse for avoiding an issue which might make you uncomfortable. *Box 2.2 contains tips on how to go about identifying children who are overweight and obese and how to raise the issue.*

Immunisations

Immunisation of children is an effective way of reducing the incidence of serious infectious diseases. No vaccine is 100% effective at protecting an individual from a disease and 'herd immunity' plays an important part in reducing their risk. All children are at higher risk of contracting the disease (whether they have been vaccinated or not) if the total uptake of the vaccine in the population is low.

If parents have not had their child vaccinated, it is worth exploring the

Box 2.2   Identifying overweight children and intervening

Identifying overweight children

Children change in shape as they grow and go through puberty. This means that different BMI values are considered normal for different ages and sexes. In order to assess whether a child is overweight, you need to plot their BMI on a UK 1990 BMI chart (use the appropriate one for their age and sex). Children whose BMI is on or above the 91st centile for their age and sex are considered overweight and those on or above the 98th centile obese (National Collaborating Centre for Primary Care and the Centre for Public Health Excellence 2006).

Scottish Intercollegiate Guidelines Network (SIGN) Guideline Number 115, *Management of Obesity* (Scottish Intercollegiate Guidelines Network 2010) contains useful clinical information on identifying and managing children with obesity. The guidance also contains links to the BMI charts.

Broaching the subject

Taking the chart with you with the child's BMI plotted on it may be helpful in starting the conversation with parents. Pointing out on a graph the normal range and the plot for their child's BMI will be a visual cue but may also help it feel less like a cosmetic judgement of their child's appearance and more of a medical assessment of their weight and height. Many parents will have heard of the BMI but give a simple explanation if they haven't.

What they can do

Acknowledge that maintaining a healthy lifestyle involving healthy food and regular exercise can be difficult for everyone but trying to make changes together as a family can help improve that child's health now and also in future. You can refer them to the change4life website (http:// www.nhs.uk/change4life) which is full of information for adults and their children about keeping healthy. It has a meal planner with cheap, healthy recipes which can be downloaded complete with an automatically generated shopping list to reduce the hassle of planning meals. For patients in England, is has information about local sports and activities. For Wales, Scotland and Northern Ireland there are other web-sites available for this (see Useful websites section at the end of this chapter).

You can also suggest that they visit their GP who will be able to help them further and refer them to relevant local services such as sport for kids and weight loss groups for parents too. Children's parents play an important part in providing role models for learned behaviours to do with eating and exercise and changes for the whole family will be much more effective.

reasons for this with them. You can also refer them to the NHS choices website (www.nhs.uk) which has lots of information about vaccinations, including an article entitled 'Why it's a good idea to get your child vaccinated' and a wall planner to help keep track of the vaccination schedule.

 Top Tip

A comprehensive guide for health professionals to all things relating to immunisations is the Department of Health publication *Immunisation against Infectious Disease* (Salisbury et al. 2006). It is more commonly referred to as 'The Green Book' and the most up-to-date version can be downloaded from the DH website for free at http:// www. dh.gov.uk/greenbook.

There are very few situations in which a vaccine may not be considered safe to give to a child (see Box 2.3). Vaccination is normally delayed if a child is suffering from a feverish illness at the time in order to avoid any developing symptoms of the febrile illness being blamed on the vaccine.

For more detail about which vaccines to give and which to avoid for children with different types of immunodeficiency, see the best practice statement *Immunisation of the Immunocompromised Child* published by the Royal College of Paediatrics and Child Health in 2002 (Cant et al. 2002) which can be found on its website (www.rcpch.ac.uk).

If children are given immunisations whilst inpatients in hospital or in the emergency department then you must communicate this by sending an 'unscheduled immunisation form' to the primary care trust, so that the child's health records can be updated, and also writing it in the child's RED BOOK.

Premature babies may still be in hospital 2 months after being born and it is important to give them their vaccinations when they reach 2 months of chronological age (one of the few circumstances when you don't use CORRECTED GESTATIONAL AGE for these babies). Babies who were born extremely premature (less than 28 weeks) should have continuous saturation and heart rate monitoring for 48–72 h after the vaccine is given as they are at risk of apnoeas, bradycardias or desaturations. If any of these occur then they should also remain in hospital to be monitored for their second set of vaccines at 3 months.

If a child has moved to the UK and it is unclear which vaccines they have received already, then assume that the child is unimmunised and follow the full UK schedule. There is an algorithm on the HPA website (www.hpa.org.uk) to help you with vaccination schedules for children who have recently moved to the UK and whose vaccination history is unclear.

The UK vaccination schedule

Fortunately, both for the children undergoing the vaccination schedule and the people having to give the vaccines, many different antigens can be included in a single combined vaccine. This helps to minimise the number of

Box 2.3   Contraindications to immunisation – advice adapted from 'The Green Book' (Salisbury et al 2006)

Severe allergy

■ Confirmed anaphylactic reaction to a previous vaccine – consult specialist before giving any further vaccinations

■ Children with confirmed anaphylactic allergy to egg should *not* receive flu or yellow fever vaccines (neither of these features routinely in the UK vaccine schedule).

■ Measles, mumps and rubella (MMR) vaccine is safe for the majority of children with egg allergy and can be given in normal conditions. However, in rare cases when a child has had a confirmed anaphylactic allergy to egg, discuss with specialist and consider giving vaccine in hospital

Contraindications to live vaccines

The only live vaccines given as part of the routine childhood schedule are the MMR vaccine and the rotavirus vaccine. The BCG vaccine (which immunises against tuberculosis) is also a live vaccine and is offered to babies and children in high-risk groups.

The rotavirus vaccine is only contraindicated in children with severe combined immune deficiency (SCID). In all other cases of immunosuppression the benefits are thought to outweigh the risks and the vaccine should be given.

The MMR vaccine is contraindicated in children who are immunosuppressed as it can sometimes cause severe infections in these patients. This includes:

■ children with severe primary immunodeficiency

■ children who have had organ transplants (and are on immunosuppressive drugs)

■ children who are taking high-dose systemic steroids (e.g. oral prednisolone at 2 mg/kg/day for 1 week or more or 1 mg/kg/day for 1 month or more) should not receive live vaccines for 3 months after steroids are stopped

■ children who are having treatment for cancer with radiotherapy or chemotherapy should not receive live vaccines for 6 months after treatment has stopped

■ children who have had a bone marrow transplant should not receive live vaccines for at least 1 year after stopping immunosuppressive treatment (but may need to leave it for even longer; discuss with their specialist as this is complicated)

■ children taking other immunosuppressive drugs such as azathioprine, methotrexate or cyclosporin should not receive live vaccine until 6 months after treatment has been stopped.

injections a child has to have in order to cover against lots of serious infectious diseases. For example, diphtheria, tetanus, pertussis, polio and *Haemophilus influenzae* type b can all be given as a single '5 IN 1' vaccine. This is sometimes also written as DTaP/IPV/Hib (D = diphtheria, T = tetanus, aP = acellular pertussis, IPV = inactivated polio virus, Hib = *Haemophilus influenzae* type b).

Table 2.3 shows the UK immunisation schedule and the number of needles this means at each sitting (which is usually the bit the child and their parents are most concerned about). It is worth noting that in some areas, the vaccines which were previously given at 13 months are now given at the same time as the 12-month vaccines instead of on two separate occasions.

There are a number of additional vaccines offered to children with certain conditions. The most common additional vaccines and their indications are listed below.

Bacillus Calmette–Guérin (BCG) vaccine against tuberculosis

For all babies less than 1 year living in an area of the UK where the annual incidence of tuberculosis is high (find out if your hospital is in one of these areas). Also offered to children who have not previously been vaccinated whose parents or grandparents were born in a country where the annual incidence of tuberculosis is more than 40/100,000 (you can find out the annual rates of tuberculosis in different countries on the World Health Organization website

Table 2.3 Immunisation schedule in the United Kingdom.

	Rotavirus (oral vaccine)	Diphtheria	Tetanus	Pertussus	Polio	Hib	PCV	MenC	MMR	HPV	No. of injections
2 months	•	•	•	•	•	•	•				2
3 months	•	•	•	•	•	•		•			2
4 months		•	•	•	•	•	•				2
12 months						•		•			1
13 months							•		•		2
3 years, 4 months		•	•	•	•				•		2
13–18 years		•	•		•			•			2
12–18 years old girls										•	3 doses spaced several months apart

Hib, *Haemophilus influenzae* type b; HPV, human papilloma virus; MenC, meningitis C; MMR, measles, mumps and rubella; PCV, pneumococcal conjugate vaccine.

at www.who.int) or who have lived there themselves for longer than 3 months. If the child is older than 6 then they are only given the vaccine after tuberculin testing if it is negative.

Varicella vaccine (chickenpox)
Offered to children older than 1 year whose siblings are immunosuppressed and therefore at risk of serious chickenpox infection. This gives some protection to the immunosuppressed child as it reduces their risk of contact with someone with active varicella infection.

Pneumococcal vaccine
Offers protection from pneumococcal infection for children with asplenia or splenic dysfunction (including children with sickle cell disease), those who are immunosuppressed and those with chronic medical conditions (including diabetes). Vaccination with the conjugated pneumococcal vaccine (PCV) is part of the routine schedule of immunisations for all children but those who are at increased risk of pneumococcal infection should also receive a single dose of pneumococcal polysaccharide vaccine (PPV) just after their second birthday.

Influenza vaccine
This is offered yearly to children with asplenia or splenic dysfunction and those who are immunosuppressed or have a chronic medical condition.

Hepatitis B
One dose given at, or shortly after, birth to babies born to infected mothers, followed by repeat doses at 1 and 2 months of age and a fourth at 1 year.

Babies who are born to highly infectious mothers should also be given hepatitis B immunoglobulin within 24 h of delivery. The need for this is decided based on the mother's blood results for various hepatitis B markers (see the Green Book or your hospital guidelines for more details). Children who require regular blood products (such as haemophiliacs) should also be vaccinated against hepatitis B.

Useful websites

Contact a Family: www.cafamily.org.uk – provides information about parent support groups and has a wealth of information on different medical conditions and syndromes

Family Fund: www.familyfund.org.uk – provides grants for families with disabled children

www.livingmadeeasy.org.uk – information about different kinds of specialist equipment and funding available towards purchasing

http:// www.nhs.uk/change4life – website full of tips on maintaining a healthy diet and keeping active for adults and children. Useful meal planning tool. Information on local activities only available for England

www.change4lifewales.org.uk – change4life for people living in Wales

www.takelifeon.co.uk – similar to change4life for people living in Scotland

www.getalifegetactive.com – similar to change4life for Northern Ireland

http:// www.dh.gov.uk/greenbook – Department of Health website; you can download a copy of 'The Green Book' from here which contains lots of information about immunisations

www.who.int – for information on incidence rates of infectious diseases in different countries

References

Cant A, Davies G, Finn A, et al. (2002) *Immunisation of the Immunocompromised Child. Best Practice Statement.* Royal College of Paediatrics and Child Health, London.

Health and Social Care Information Centre (2013) *Statistics on Obesity, Physical Activity and Diet: England 2013*, Health and Social Care Information Centre, Leeds.

Innocenti Research Centre (2007) *Promoting the Rights of Children with Disabilities.* Innocenti Digest No. 13. UNICEF Innocenti Research Centre, Florence.

National Collaborating Centre for Primary Care and the Centre for Public Health Excellence (2006) *Obesity. Guidance on the Prevention, Identification, Assessment and Management of Overweight and Obesity in Adults and Children.* NICE Clinical Guideline No. 43. National Institute for Health and Clinical Excellence, London.

Salisbury D, Ramsay M, Noakes K (2006) *Immunisation against Infectious Disease.* Stationery Office, Norwich.

Scottish Intercollegiate Guidelines Network (2010) *Management of Obesity.* Scottish Intercollegiate Guidelines Network, Edinburgh.

Chapter 3
COMMUNICATION WITH CHILDREN AND THEIR PARENTS

Communication with children and their parents presents all sorts of unique challenges. Most doctors in the early stages of their career will not be parents themselves and may have very little experience of communicating with children. This can lead to the temptation to simply talk about the child to their parents. Children can find this very frustrating, particularly as they get older, and understandably so. Involve the child in the consultation as much as you can; it is after all their health you are discussing. How much they are able to contribute will vary according to their age, maturity and confidence but you should always give them plenty of opportunities to talk.

Communicating well is a skill which takes a lot of practice and sometimes even the most experienced and able communicators don't get it quite right. This chapter aims to arm you with some initial hints and tricks, but the only way you will really learn is through trying out different things to find out what works for you and what doesn't.

Some key points to stick to whatever the child's age include the following.

■ **Be honest**. Don't say it's not going to hurt if it will as this undermines the child's trust in you.

■ **Explain in simple terms, but not too simple**. Choose a level of detail that is suitable for the child's age. Pictures can help to explain things to people of all ages and role play with puppets can be helpful for younger children. It can be difficult to get the level of detail in your explanations right. You don't want to oversimplify what you are saying as this can be enormously frustrating for children as they hate being patronised but you do want them to understand clearly what you are telling them. Establishing their level of understanding first can be very helpful in judging what sort of explanation will be appropriate.

■ **Take the child seriously**. It is really important for children of all ages to feel that they are important and worth listening to. Listen to what they have to tell you and take them seriously. Try to talk *with* them, not *at* them and avoid being patronising.

■ **Move to the child's level**. If you're both sitting on chairs in clinic then this is

The Hands-on Guide to Practical Paediatrics, First Edition. Rebecca Hewitson and Caroline Fertleman.
© 2014 John Wiley & Sons, Ltd. Published 2014 by John Wiley & Sons, Ltd.
Companion Website: www.wileyhandsonguides.com/paediatrics

easier; if not, then crouch down so that you are talking to them at their own level, or even sit down on the floor.

■ **Sit them nearest to you**. Having the child rather than their parent in the seat nearest to you makes it clear who is the focus of the consultation. You wouldn't ever see an adult patient and sit the relative next to you and the patient further away so don't do it with children either. Very young children may not be able to cope with this due to a fear of strangers but children from 3 years and older should be comfortable with this set-up.

■ **Eye contact**. Look at the child and address questions directly to them, rather than talking across them to their parent.

■ **Focus on the child first**. Go to collect them from the waiting room and address the child first, introducing yourself. You can then start your consultation by asking the child who they have brought with them to see you. This puts the focus immediately on them rather than their parents or carers.

■ **Be flexible**. Knowing a child's age will give you a rough idea of what to expect but children do vary enormously in terms of their level of maturity and how confident they are at expressing themselves. Be alert to the child's body language and tone of voice and if your initial approach is not working, try something different.

■ **Be pleased to see them**. It doesn't matter how busy or stressed you are, it is vital that the child feels that you have time and are happy to see them. If not, then they will not feel welcome and may

not have the confidence to speak to you at all. A genuinely warm welcome, a smile and using their first name when greeting them can help the child to feel comfortable.

■ **Begin with something easy to talk about**. Launching straight into what the problem is doesn't help children to feel like talking. Try beginning with a non-threatening topic first. This will vary depending on the age of the child and what is happening for them in their life at the time – school can be an obvious topic that seems safe to talk about but if they have missed a lot of school because of their health, the child may not want to talk to you about it. Look at the age-specific examples below but also watch what their response is and change the topic if you are getting nowhere.

■ **Don't forget to briefly acknowledge any other children**. Children may often come to consultations with their siblings. It is important to briefly greet any other children too and provide appropriate toys for them to play with to avoid distraction. Seeing their

 Top Tip

It is particularly important to involve disabled children in discussions as much as they are able. They often feel ignored and underestimated in many different aspects of their lives so showing that you want to listen to them is enormously important and will be very much appreciated by their parents too.

older sibling interacting with you can help younger children to have the confidence to speak to you.

How to communicate with a baby or toddler

Don't forget that even before children are able to talk, they can still be very expressive and can understand some of what you are saying (the tone of conversation if not all of the content). Babies and toddlers will often be wary of new people and may be very shy or upset.

■ **Talk to the child first**. Although they will not be able to contribute to giving you a history of their illness, it is important to talk to the child initially to help to establish their trust and also because parents find it very disconcerting if you completely ignore their child.

■ **Make a positive comment about the child**. With babies and toddlers, it can be helpful to greet them at the very beginning of the consultation and briefly comment on a toy they have with them or an item of clothing. For example, you can point at a cuddly toy they may have and ask 'Who's this? He looks like a very friendly teddy bear' or 'Wow, I love your bright blue shoes'. You are unlikely to get any response from the child but this is not the aim; you are just trying to make them more comfortable and to demonstrate to their parents that you really are child centred. Keep it brief before moving on to

discussion with the parents and providing appropriate toys for the child to play with whilst you do this.

Top Tip

It can be helpful to carry a small toy with you to entertain very young children. Brightly coloured and highly contrasting toys are often the most effective. Make sure that it is made of a material that can withstand being cleaned with alcohol wipes and that there are no small parts that could end up being choked on.

■ **'Examine' a toy or parent first**. Very young children have a short attention span and learn through playing. To make examination less threatening, it can be helpful to examine them on their parent's lap and to start by examining their parent or cuddly toy first and engage the child in helping you to do so. When you start examining the child, start by placing the stethoscope on their hand first as this is much less threatening than immediately placing it on their chest.

■ **Try whispering**. Sometimes, even with the greatest efforts on your part a young child will begin to cry as soon as you try to examine them. You can try going back to examining the parent or cuddly toy a little more first or sometimes whispering or talking very quietly to them can help as they become so fixed on trying to hear what you are saying that they settle a little and become less fearful.

How to communicate with an infant school child (4–6 years)

By the time a child reaches school age, they will often be able to contribute to the consultation and give some of the history for themselves. There can be a wide variation in maturity, though, and whilst some children of this age may be very chatty and confident, others may say virtually nothing.

■ **Start with easy topics** such as what they like to do when they're not at school, what they were playing with in the waiting room or what their favourite television programme is; this can be helpful in building their trust and encouraging them to talk. It will also help you to establish how much the child is likely to be able to relay details of the history themselves.

■ **Try asking the child what's happening first.** You can start by asking the child an open question about why they have come to see you and try to gain some of the basic history from them. In all cases you probably need to clarify some of the details with the parents and how soon you do this will depend on how confident the child is about telling you what is going on themselves.

■ **Acknowledge the child's contribution before talking with parents.** When switching to talking to their parents instead, the child needs to feel that their input has been important and that you are not ignoring what they have told you. Helpful expressions might include 'Thank you for telling me that, I'd like to hear what your mum/dad thinks about all this too'.

■ **Don't forget about the child.** Once you have started talking to the parent, don't forget to occasionally direct questions to the child too rather than simply taking the rest of the history from the parent.

■ **Clarify words and phrases used.** It can be helpful to clarify with the parents some of the language that their child uses for certain pieces of anatomy or bodily functions and use these words yourself when talking to the child.

How to communicate with a school-age child (7–12 years)

By this age many children will be able to tell you most of their medical history themselves. Sitting the child on the chair nearest to you and their parent on the one furthest away helps to show who you expect to be doing most of the talking. Many children of this age will respond well to being treated more like an adult; consider shaking their hand as they come in first and then their parent's hand too as you introduce yourself.

■ **Find out what the child wants.** As part of taking a history from the child, it is important to find out more about how they feel about their illness and what they would like to be done about it. One way of finding out more about the child's hopes and fears can be by asking a question such as 'If I could magically grant you three wishes, what would you wish for?' or 'If we could change one thing about your illness, what would it be?'. This can help to establish what is important for that child, which may be being able to play football with their friends or not having to take medications whilst they are at school.

 Top Tip

From around 7 years onwards, many children can benefit from having a chance to talk to their doctor without their parents present. After you have had an initial discussion with the child and their parents, you can explain to them that your routine practice is to allow the child to discuss things directly with you without their parents present. This allows you to establish trust with the child and the parents first so that they feel more comfortable with the idea. You can tell the child that you won't discuss anything they tell you with their parents or anyone else, unless you are worried that they are being harmed in some way in which case you may have to. It can be useful to establish with the child what you will discuss with their parents and what you will not before you invite the parents back into the room. You can encourage children to discuss issues with their parents but do not breach their right to confidentiality by sharing this information yourself unless you need to for the child's safety or welfare.

■ **Work on a solution together**. Once you have established what is important to them, you can then work on coming up with a solution together. You can try asking things like 'What do you think we should do about this?' or 'What can we do together to make this happen?'. Involving the child in decision making about treatment options is important for helping them to feel in control of what is happening.

 Top Tip

Confidence and maturity vary a lot between different children of the same age and you must adjust your consultation accordingly for each individual child. Bear in mind that when a child is acutely unwell, they are likely to regress to behaviour that would be typical of a younger child. It may be that in the acute situation, the parent will give you more of the history than you would normally expect for a child of that age. Once the child is more stable and feeling better, you can take time to go back and talk to them in more detail about their illness and what has happened as they will be much more able and willing to interact with you at this stage.

How to communicate with a teenager

For more information about specific issues affecting teenagers, such as sexual and mental health, see Chapter 8 – Teenagers.

Consultations with teenagers can be some of the most challenging to get right and doctors sometimes feel quite intimidated at the prospect of trying to talk to a teenager. Adolescence is a time of many changes both physically and behaviourally and these stages of development happen at different ages for different people. Recent research into the developing brain has found that certain areas of the brain (such as the prefrontal cortex) undergo significant changes during adolescence (Mills et al. 2012). The prefrontal cortex is involved in self-awareness, inhibition (particularly of risk-taking behaviour) and our ability to understand other people and how their perspectives might differ from our own. Understanding this can help you to realise that some of the stereotypical behaviours associated with adolescence, such as risk taking or failing to see things from someone else's perspective, are actually a normal part of neurodevelopment.

Adolescence is also a time of forming an adult personality and establishing more independence from parents and caregivers. Part of this process often involves rebellion of some kind or challenging of authority figures in order to assert independence. This can be particularly problematic for teenagers who are unwell and as a consequence have become more dependent on others for care.

Some general rules that may help during discussions with teenagers include the following.

■ **Be yourself**. Honesty and openness from doctors can be enormously reassuring for teenagers so being genuine can really help to establish trust. This means, whatever you do, don't try to be cool; it will not go down well and you will probably come across as false or difficult to take seriously.

■ **Be interested in them as a person**. Start off the consultation by asking about their life (school, personal interests, part-time jobs, etc.) and be genuinely interested in what they have to say. Listen actively and follow up with further questions about things that they have mentioned, picking up on cues within what they say to talk more about topics they enjoy. This initial conversation can be useful in redressing the balance of power by allowing them to tell you about something you know nothing about. For example, if they mention something that you have never heard of, ask them more about it and have a short conversation about whatever it is.

■ **Don't tell, ask**. In our desire to help and anxiety about filling awkward silences, it can be all too easy for a consultation to turn into you giving a mini-lecture. This unsolicited advice can be resented as it makes the teenager feel that you are being patronising and don't care about what they have to say. Telling people what to do rarely changes their behaviour; instead, ask questions to find out more about how their illness is affecting them, what they are hoping to be able to achieve and what frustrations they have with the way things currently are. This can help you to come up with a management plan based on a shared agreement rather than simply a list of things coming from you that is likely to be ignored. Ask questions like 'If you could change one thing about your illness, what would it be?', 'How can we work together to achieve that?' and 'What annoys you about your illness/ treatment?' to find out what they want.

■ **Empower them to make changes**. Teenagers can be far more resourceful and creative than adults and are often able to find novel solutions to problems that you would never have thought of yourself. Encouraging them to come up with their own ideas for how to deal with their illness and its treatment can allow them to make meaningful changes.

■ **Ask, don't assume you know**. Poor compliance with medications and treatments is a common problem when dealing with adolescent patients and there are many possible underlying reasons. It may be that the patient is finding it difficult to remember to take their medication or that it is a deliberate choice not to. This is not just a teenage problem; many adults also have trouble complying with medications and acknowledging this can be helpful. They may simply have trouble remembering to take their medications and working through ideas with them for how they might remember would be helpful. Maybe they are refusing to take their medication as a way of rebelling against authority figures (you and their parents) or they don't see any possible negative consequences of not taking it. It may also be that they are concerned about the side-effects of medications and what to do if these happen and they want an explanation of these and where to go for help if they do occur.

■ **Offer information and choices**. Provide teenagers with plenty of information about the options that are available to them and explain the reasons why you think a particular medication or treatment may be helpful for them. You can suggest a list of possible options of what to do and ask them which one they would like. This may be offering a choice of medications with different side-effect profiles, discussing what would happen if no treatment is started or agreeing to a trial period of a particular treatment before you meet again to see how it is working. This allows them to make informed decisions about their own health. *For more about consent see Consent section later in this chapter and Chapter 8 – Teenagers.*

■ **Focus on them, not on their illness**. Try to keep the consultation focused on them as an individual and ways in which their illness affects their life. Telling a teenager that they need to take a particular medication because it says so in a guideline or protocol is not helpful. Talk instead about how certain treatments or medications could alter the symptoms they have told you about and help them to get around some of the problems that they have mentioned. Avoid making assumptions about how their illness limits them if possible and how they view themselves. It may be that they see themselves as being very well (despite your own perception of their health) and their illness or DISABILITY has a minimal impact on them.

■ **Be totally non-judgemental**. It can be very difficult for teenagers to open up about things that they find embarrassing and to talk about behaviours that they think are going to get them into trouble. Be aware of your own facial expressions and make sure that you don't appear shocked or disgusted by what they are telling you as this will rapidly discourage them from talking. Normalising certain behaviours can sometimes be a useful way of encouraging them to talk; for example, 'A lot of people your age drink alcohol; do any of your friends drink?'. Starting by asking about friends first can be useful before asking them about themselves.

■ **See them without their parents present**. It is important to give teenagers an opportunity to talk to you independently, without their parents present. They value privacy and may feel able to share things with you that they would not be comfortable saying if their parents were present. It can be helpful to explain this process at the beginning of the consultation with teenagers and point out that this is part of your normal practice so that parents understand why they are being asked to leave the room. Talking to parents and teenagers about confidentiality is also important so that they know what to expect. Explain that anything that the teenager tells you will remain in confidence unless you are worried that they are being harmed in some way, in which case you are obliged to share it with some other people who need to know (for example, with other doctors or their parents) but that you will explain to the teenager exactly what you are telling to whom before you do so. After you have talked to the teenager on their own, it can be useful to agree

with them what you are going to share with their parents and what you are not. You can encourage teenagers to share information about what you have discussed with their parents but must never disclose information unless you have their permission. If you have concerns about the teenager's welfare, it can be helpful to discuss with senior colleagues or a named child protection nurse or doctor to get their advice before deciding what to disclose to parents.

■ **Be aware of your own feelings**. It is natural within conversations to subconsciously mirror certain behaviour and body language. This can be very helpful for establishing rapport and is entirely appropriate at times but there are certain instances when it can be unhelpful. For example, if a teenager is very angry or hostile it can be difficult to remain warm and engaged in your own behaviour because their anger can invoke a lot of angry feelings in you. Awareness of your own feelings and body language can be helpful when a consultation is not going well. Similarly, if a teenager is trying to avoid talking about a certain issue you might pick up on these cues and avoid asking these important questions. Be brave and have the courage to ask about difficult subjects.

■ **If the conversation is going badly, acknowledge it and apologise**. Sometimes, a consultation can start badly and then it feels difficult to get things back on track. Sometimes acknowledging this by talking about it can help rescue a conversation that is not going well. For example, saying something like 'I'm sorry, we seem to have got off to a bad start, I'm talking too much and really

I'm interested to hear what you have to say'. This can make you seem more human and approachable by admitting your mistake and can allow a renewed attempt to have a useful conversation.

How to communicate with a child using alternative communication

For many children with learning difficulties, physical or sensory IMPAIRMENT, communication with others can be difficult, but it is crucial that they are given the support to do so. Children who have difficulty speaking may use alternative and augmentative communication (AAC). AAC is the overarching term used to describe a number of different ways of communicating.

■ **Communication charts and symbol boards**. The child will point at different symbols to communicate or use letter boards to spell out individual words in some cases.

■ **Electronic equipment** such as voice synthesisers (sometimes known as voice output communication aids).

■ **Signing**, gesture or symbol-based languages.

If you have no previous experience of working with people who use AAC to communicate then it can feel quite daunting at first knowing what to do. There are learning modules available on the Scope website (www.scope.org.uk) about AAC. Another useful resource is *Other Ways of Speaking*, a booklet about communicating with children who are using AAC. It is published by the Communication Trust and available to download free from their website (www.thecommunicationtrust.org.uk). The following pieces of advice are adapted from these two resources.

■ **Admit if you are uncertain**. It can be very helpful to tell the child and their parents if this is the first time you have met someone who uses AAC to communicate. This will allow them to show you their method of communicating at the beginning and make the whole process much easier.

■ **Establish 'yes' and 'no'**. Ask at the beginning of the consultation how the child communicates 'yes' and 'no'. This may be different from the nod and shake of the head that you were expecting. For example, a child may smile for 'yes' and look down for 'no'.

■ **Be patient**. It is important to give children time to respond to your question as it may take them much longer than other people to be able to answer. It is frustrating if you ask them a question and then turn to their parent for an answer rather than giving them time to answer for themselves.

■ **Pick up non-verbal cues**. Facial expressions and body language can be even more important in communicating a child's feelings if they are using AAC so pay attention to these.

■ **Talk at eye level**. Just as you would with any other child, get down to their level and look at them when you are talking to them, not at their communication aid or their carers.

■ **Don't talk about the child.** In exactly the same way as you would in a consultation with any other child, don't simply talk about them with their parents without acknowledging the fact that you are doing this, e.g. 'I'd like to hear what your dad has to say about things too'.

■ **Clarify if you don't understand.** It is important not to pretend that you have understood what the child is trying to tell you if you haven't. Give them the opportunity to clarify what they meant so that you can understand them properly.

■ **Allow plenty of time.** It can take a lot longer to have conversations with children using AAC so try to set aside plenty of time. If you are short on time, then explain this at the beginning of the consultation and agree to come back later.

■ **Summarise.** At the end of the conversation, summarise what you have talked about and check that you have interpreted everything correctly. Give the child time to clarify any misunderstandings.

How to communicate with anxious parents

Many doctors will say that before they became parents themselves, they never really appreciated quite how scary it is when your child is unwell, even when you are armed with far more knowledge than the general population. Parents tend to be much more anxious about their child's health than they would be about their own because of the responsibility of having to interpret how the child is feeling, fear of being a bad parent if they don't seek help early and sometimes because of social factors (such as grandparents expressing concern or being unsupported at home).

Whilst it is certainly true that some people are more prone to worrying than others, it is important to avoid simply labelling someone as an 'anxious parent' at your first meeting. This can be really unhelpful for them, their child and for you for the following reasons.

■ **Parents still worried.** Even if you offer reassurance that their child is well, unless you have addressed their specific concerns the parents may still leave feeling just as anxious as they did before.

■ **Parents reluctant to return.** If you have told them that their child is fine and not seemed to appreciate why they were concerned then the parents may assume that they were overreacting and will not seek help again if the child becomes more unwell, meaning that the child does not get medical attention when they really need it.

■ **You may miss important clinical information.** If you have already convinced yourself that there is nothing really wrong with the child and the parent is simply an 'anxious parent', you may overlook vital clues in the history that point towards a particular pathology.

■ **They may lose trust in you.** Sometimes, particularly if you see a child very early on in the natural progression of an illness, they will appear well but may subsequently deteriorate. This can undermine your own confidence in your diagnostic abilities and leave you wondering if you missed something. In reality, it is impossible to predict what will happen sometimes and it may be that your decision was entirely reasonable based on the child's condition at that time. The problem is that parents will probably not see it that way, particularly if they felt you hadn't properly listened to them at the initial consultation or explained that you were happy to see them again if things changed.

Avoiding the trap of dismissing parents as just being 'anxious' is half the battle. Once you have managed that, here are some suggestions for making sure that you fully address their concerns.

■ **Find out the social context**. Are they isolated and lacking support? Do they have grandparents or friends interfering and telling them that their child is very unwell? Has someone in their family recently died or been given a serious diagnosis? All these things can contribute to raised anxiety levels.

■ **Ask about specific concerns**. It can be useful to address the issue outright rather than skirting around it. Obviously, this requires you to phrase things well, as 'Why are you worried?' doesn't sound very supportive and can make people defensive. Instead, ask something like 'Is there anything in particular that you're worried is going on here?'. It's amazing what you can find out by asking this question. Parents will often feel reluctant to volunteer their thoughts as they think that you as the doctor are

supposed to be the one making a diagnosis, but asking directly gives them permission to tell you. Without addressing these specifics, you are unable to really provide any reassurance that is helpful.

■ **Explain your reasoning**. Talking parents through the specifics of why you have decided to do what you are doing can help a lot. If nothing else, then it shows them that you are actually taking time to think about what to do, which is reassuring in itself. It can also be empowering for them to understand some of the factors behind the decision that you are making and shows that you have listened to what they have told you.

■ **Don't forget your safety net**. It is important that parents know when to come back for help so be as specific as you can. For example, 'If your child is getting more unwell, come back' isn't helpful as they thought that the child was unwell now but you think they are safe to go home. This advice is only helpful if it is backed up with some specific examples and a time frame too; for example, 'If he becomes drowsy, isn't wetting as many nappies as normal or his symptoms aren't improving in the next two or three days then come back'.

How to communicate with an expert parent or patient

Children with long-term conditions and their parents often become experts on their particular condition. In fact, they may have more knowledge on the subject than you do, particularly if their condition is a rare one. Given the amount of information now available on the internet, it is possible for patients to be very well informed before they come to see the doctor. This can be a difficult relationship to manage as a junior doctor as you may feel the need to prove yourself and your level of knowledge to the patient and their parents in an attempt to reassure yourself about your own level of competence.

■ **Acknowledge their expertise**. It is important to acknowledge how much they know about the topic, not just by saying that but also with your actions and the way that you run the consultation.

■ **Don't assume expertise**. You may come across parents who are healthcare professionals or scientists and feel that you should talk to them differently from other parents. However, it may be the case that they don't know much about this particular area and what they do know is likely to be forgotten in the stressful context of being the parent of a child who is unwell. They may be too embarrassed to ask for clarification of things that they don't understand as they feel that they ought to know. It can be helpful to acknowledge their job but explain that you are going to start out by treating them just the same as any other parent. This can be an enormous relief for some parents as it allows them to be free of their healthcare role and concentrate solely on being a parent.

■ **Find out what they want from you**. Given that they are much more informed about their condition, it is

unlikely that these patients are coming to you for a diagnosis or for basic information about their disease and you will need to take a different approach. Starting the consultation with something like 'What can I help you with today?' can be a good way of finding out what they want to discuss with you.

■ **Admit the limits of your own knowledge**. You undermine the patient's trust in you and can end up looking very foolish if you pretend to know more than you actually do. Fully admit when you do not know the answer, but look into ways of helping the patient despite this.

■ **Offer to find out more**. You need to admit when you don't know the answer yourself but can offer to look up more information in the medical literature and discuss with colleagues with specialist expertise. Establish when and how you will communicate this information to them; it may be that arranging a follow-up consultation is the most useful way of doing this.

■ **Find out their concerns and hopes**. This is important in allowing you to find out relevant information. It's all very well you looking up the latest research on medications that reduce the number of hospital admissions but if all your patient is worried about is the side-effect profiles then you will not be able to help them. It also allows the conversation to still be a useful one for the patient and their parents in giving them space to discuss how their illness is affecting their life and what they were hoping to be able to change. Even if you don't have the relevant knowledge at that time, you can use your listening skills to make the consultation a success.

Breaking bad news

When people think of breaking bad news, their initial thought is often of parents being told that their child has died. In reality, this shouldn't be something you have to do as a junior member of the team. However, there are so many other types of bad news that we have to break to parents and sometimes the challenge can be recognising it as bad news in the first place.

We become very accustomed to being around people who are ill, we know a lot about the symptoms of diseases and their treatment and come across great examples of people with long-term conditions who are able to manage their illness so that it has a minimal impact on their life. This can sometimes make us a little blind to how it feels for parents to be told that their child has a condition that they know nothing about. Or even worse, being told that their child has a condition that they have seen someone close to them die of (for example, parents are sometimes terrified when you tell them that their child has pneumonia as they may have had an elderly relative who died of pneumonia and they think that their child is going to die too).

'Bad news' isn't just telling someone about a cancer diagnosis or death; it is a very subjective reaction to a wide variety of topics so always be alert to how a child and parent are reacting to what you are telling them. Try to mirror how

they are reacting – you don't want to be talking very gravely about something that they hadn't really thought was an issue or being cheerful and matter of fact about something which they think is terrible news.

There are some pieces of bad news that should only really be broken to parents by a senior member of the team with experience in doing so. Do not tell the parents yourself before consulting with your senior colleagues in the following instances.

■ **Inherited conditions**. This can be associated with a lot of guilt for some parents that they have passed on an illness to their child. It can also have implications for any further children they were planning to have as well as their child's ability to have a family of their own.

■ **Developmental delay or disability**. It can be very distressing for parents to hear that their child has some form of IMPAIRMENT or DEVELOPMENTAL DELAY. The way in which the news is broken is very important and this must be done sensitively and the person telling them must know enough about the condition to be able to answer their questions. Scope, a charity that works with disabled children and their families, has developed guidance on how news should be broken to parents about their child having additional needs (whether that be a physical or sensory impairment, learning or behavioural difficulties). Its 'Right from the Start' best practice guidelines can be found on its website (www.scope.org.uk).

■ **Long-term conditions**. Telling a child and their parents that they have an illness that will be with them for the rest of their life is a big deal. For example, to you asthma and diabetes may be easily treatable conditions and not something to be overly worried about. However, for the child and the parent this is something that will affect the entirety of the rest of their lives: attending clinic appointments, remembering to take medications and worrying about what school friends will think.

■ **Needing an operation**. This is a scary thing for a parent and child to be told. There are lots of uncertainties, they may be worried about pain or complications of surgery, whether or not it will work, who the surgeon will be. It takes an enormous amount of trust in the medical team from the parent and child to undergo a surgical procedure, no matter how minor. They are totally reliant on the skills of people, some of whom they will never have met who are going to knock them unconscious and take a scalpel to their skin. This is a daunting prospect for any child or parent.

■ **Any problem that is irreversible**. This can be anything from finding that the child has congenital deafness to brain damage after a head injury.

The following are also examples of 'bad news' but it may be appropriate for you to discuss these with parents yourself.

■ **Delayed investigations/treatment**. For you, this might seem like a minor inconvenience, but telling a family that a planned investigation or treatment is going to be delayed can actually be received as terrible news. The child may have been feeling anxious about what is going to happen and this prolongs their feeling of apprehension. The parents might be concerned about how this will impact on the child's health. Will it damage their child's health to delay the treatment? Could more be done if the results of an investigation are available sooner? It also makes it very difficult for parents who have other children. They may need to leave the hospital to collect their other children from school and will feel torn between their responsibility to their other children and the child who is in hospital.

■ **Being told that your new baby is anything less than perfect**. The birth of a new baby is an incredibly emotional time for parents. Their expectation is that this new baby is going to be completely normal and healthy so if this is not the case then this is very bad news (even if the problem seems minor to you). If the baby is unwell and has to be separated from the mother to receive treatment, this separation can cause a lot of distress to the mother. A helpful source of advice and support for parents of premature and sick babies is the Best Beginnings charity (www.bestbeginnings.org.uk).

■ **Being told that your child needs to be admitted to hospital**. This is stressful news, regardless of the cause. Hospitals are not nice places to be and the very fact that the child is unwell enough to need admission can cause worry. Also, the child being admitted to the ward can cause major disruption to the parents' lives and that of their other children.

■ **Anything that is badly timed or will restrict future activities**. The news itself may be bad because of its timing, for example, that the treatment for an illness is going to clash with important exams for the child or that as a result of their discovered colour blindness, a teenager will have to give up their dream of becoming a pilot.

Having to break bad news to parents is something that most doctors dread but is so important to get right. Whole books have been written on this topic and it is a skill that takes a lot of practice. Charities such as Child Bereavement UK run courses on breaking bad news, providing support for families who have been bereaved or who have children with life-limiting conditions or complex needs. This charity also has lots of useful learning resources on its website and a support helpline for professionals and for family members (www. childbereavementuk.org).

Here are some suggestions for making sure that you break the bad news well.

■ **Talk to the parents without the child present first**. This is different from normal consultations when you talk with the parents and the child simultaneously. However, it is important to give the parents the opportunity to talk to you alone first. This means that they don't have to put on a 'brave face' in order to avoid upsetting or scaring their child and can ask questions that they may not feel comfortable asking with their child present. It also allows them to decide how much information they will share with younger children

about their illness and where and how they will go about doing this.

■ **Have all the relevant people present**. If both parents are involved in caring for the child, it is really important for both of them to be present whenever you are breaking bad news in order for them to be a support to each other but also so that the information that they receive is the same. For single parents, they may wish to have other people present instead, such as a friend or a relative. You can arrange this by saying that you need to have an important conversation with them and arranging a time to do this, before asking if there is anyone who they would like to have with them at the time. This may not always be possible, for example if a child is needing immediate admission to hospital, but if you have any opportunity to plan how and when to break bad news, make every effort to ensure that all the relevant people are present.

■ **Somewhere private and sitting down**. Don't break bad news in a corridor or other public place. Breaking of bad news should be done in a separate room with the door closed. Make sure that you and both of the parents are able to sit down. Standing up makes it seem like you are going to leave at any moment, whereas sitting down gives a clear message that you will take time to listen to them and puts you on the same eye level which is important.

■ **Take a colleague with you**. It can be really helpful to have another colleague with you whilst you are breaking bad news, to help support the family. For example, having a nurse there who has been caring for the child can be very helpful for parents and can help make the situation feel slightly less daunting for you.

■ **Read up beforehand**. You need to be as confident as possible about the information you are relaying so that you can answer any questions that the parents may have as fully as possible. Anxiety about the subject matter can get in the way of your ability to communicate effectively so feeling confident about this part is important. Admit when you don't know the answer to a question, but offer to find out and get back to them.

■ **Avoid interruptions**. Ask someone else to hold your bleep and make sure that your mobile phone is switched off if you have it with you. Tell colleagues which room you are using and why and ask them not to disturb you.

■ **Find out how much they already know**. It is important to establish what they already think is going on and if they have had any suspicions or worries about potential diagnoses. This helps you to know where to start with your explanation.

■ **Avoid using jargon**. A defence mechanism that doctors sometimes use to protect themselves from upsetting situations is to resort to using medical jargon. This is really unhelpful for families who may be irritated by you using unfamiliar words or completely misinterpret what you are trying to tell them. Explain using simple language only, except to name the diagnosis. It is important that families know the technical name for the diagnosis, so do give them this but follow with an explanation of what it means.

■ **Empathy**. Showing concern and understanding can make a big difference to how bad news is received. Everyone has their own way of showing empathy but the underlying sentiment is the important part. Try to understand and accept the family's feelings and viewpoints and be sensitive to their body language and your own. Maintaining eye contact can promote trust. Use phrases that acknowledge what they appear to be feeling; for example, 'I can see this has come as quite a shock' or 'I understand that this is very upsetting for you'.

■ **Be prepared for a wide range of reactions**. There is an enormous variety in the range of responses different people will have to the same news and it is important to be prepared for any of these to happen. Bad news can be met with different responses such as anger, denial, tears or shock.

■ **Don't treat tears as an emergency that need to be stopped**. It's great to be thoughtful and offer a tissue if a patient is crying but thrusting the whole box in their face in an urgent manner can seem like an attempt to stop the crying. The best thing to do can just be to sit in silence with them whilst they cry. Touching their hand or arm can show support without the need to say anything if you feel comfortable doing this, but be aware that in some cultures (such as religious Muslims or Jews), you should not touch parents of the opposite gender.

■ **Don't leave the room or run off**. It is really uncomfortable telling people bad news and this can leave you with the urge to get out of the situation as quickly as possible. It is really important to fight this and make yourself stay with the family rather than running off at the earliest opportunity. Families really notice this and showing that you have time for them and are comfortable being with them whilst they are upset can make a big difference.

■ **Allow time for parents to ask you questions**. Parents may have questions they want to ask and it is important that you offer them this opportunity. It may be that they are unable to think of anything after the initial shock of hearing the news, in which case you can offer to meet with them again later once they have had a chance for it to sink in.

■ **Expect to have to give the information more than once**. Sometimes doctors will express frustration that after a lengthy conversation with parents about the child's illness, they later ask the same questions that have already been discussed. This is not necessarily a reflection on the quality of the explanation you have given them and should not be taken personally. It is to be expected that parents will not be able to remember everything from the first consultation, particularly if you have told them bad news. Often patients and parents will report remembering next to nothing of what was said after the bad news was shared with them. Breaking down the information into small chunks at the time can help with this but it is to be expected that you will have to repeat most information at least a second time.

■ **Give time for decisions to be made**. It takes time for parents to come to terms with what you have told them; they may need several explanations before they can retain the information and may only think of important questions after they have had time to think. It is therefore important to allow plenty of time for parents to make decisions about their child's care if this is possible.

■ **Offer support in telling their children the news**. One of the big concerns that parents can have when they have been told bad news about their child is to know how much to tell them and how to go about it. It is important for children to be informed (even if only on a simple level) about what is happening otherwise their parents' upset can be very confusing to them and they can feel very angry and hurt about being left out. Offering support to parents in sharing news with their children (including any siblings) can be a source of great comfort. Breaking bad news to children is very tricky to do well and may be best left to a senior colleague or done with the involvement of a play specialist for young children. If you do have to break bad news to a child, always do so with their parents present, find out what they already know (children are very perceptive and may already have picked up a great deal more about what is happening than you had realised), explain in simple terms and find out what they are worried or scared about after you have told them. It is important to explain to them that the illness is nobody's fault as children may often see the disease as a punishment for bad behaviour.

Cultural sensitivity

This can be a very difficult thing to get right. It is important to be aware of certain cultural differences and alter your practice accordingly to be sensitive to the family's needs. However, it is also crucial to avoid stereotyping and assuming that individuals hold the same views as others from a similar cultural or ethnic background. Here are some suggestions to consider during your practice.

■ **Find out their individual views.** Treating each patient and their families as individuals is very important so avoid making assumptions. It is perfectly possible for a doctor and patient who are from the same ethnic and cultural background to have entirely different opinions and the doctor making assumptions about that individual's values and beliefs can cause offence or misunderstanding. Keeping a focus on the patient and family in front of you and establishing their own ideas and values can help to overcome some of this. Treat your patients and their families as individuals, rather than as members of a cultural group.

■ **Use a professional translator.** Even patients whose English is quite good may miss some of the subtleties of what you are trying to tell them (and vice versa) unless you have the help of a translator. Children are much more likely to speak both English and their mother tongue fluently and it is tempting to use them as a translator. However, this places an unfair burden on the child and can end up with information being withheld or misinterpreted. It is much better to use a professional translator, either in person or using one of the telephone translation services that are available from many hospitals.

■ **Ask how they prefer to be addressed.** It is really important to address people correctly and establish the correct pronunciation of their name. No matter how daunting it may seem, always attempt to pronounce the name yourself to show that you are willing to make the effort and appear interested and if possible continue to use their name throughout the consultation. Don't make assumptions about the names of different family members as this will vary between cultures and between individual preferences. The mother and father may have different surnames but they may still be married as many women choose to keep their original name and some cultures have an entirely different system of names. Clarify which is their formal name and which is their familiar name as the order in which these are written also differs between cultures.

■ **Ask where the child was born.** Finding out where the child was born is important in establishing their social background. This gives information about whether this is a child who was born elsewhere and has had to adapt to a new life or if they have been born and brought up in the same place. It can also be helpful to find out where parents were born too for the same reasons.

■ **Learn about different cultures.** Learning a little bit about other cultures can be helpful in allowing you to anticipate some of the possible views and practices of individuals from that community. This can be done through discussion with patients, but it is also advisable to do a little background reading, focusing on cultures that predominate in the population that your hospital serves. For example, if you know that there is a substantial Muslim population living in your area, it may be useful to find out more about key religious beliefs and customs in relation to healthcare held by this religion. It is possible to use this knowledge in a helpful way, without making assumptions about the patient, by asking questions. For example, 'I know that some people of the Muslim faith will be fasting at this time of year; is this the case for you?'.

■ **If you don't know, ask**. You may come across customs and practices that you are not familiar with and if this is the case then ask. It is far better to clarify than to make assumptions and as long as you ask in a respectful way, people will usually be pleased that you are showing an interest in wanting to understand more about their culture.

■ **Children may feel torn between two cultures**. It can be useful to recognise that some children may struggle with conflicting ideas between different cultures in which they have grown up: that of their parents and that of their school friends from different cultural backgrounds. It may sometimes be tempting to offer an opinion but this can often result in you making assumptions based on your own cultural background and can be unhelpful for the child. Instead, encourage them to talk about some of the things that they are struggling with and listen to what they

have to say, helping them to come up with their own solutions rather than offering advice.

■ **Consider involving other colleagues**. You may be able to seek advice from colleagues who are from a similar cultural background to that of your patient. They may be able to explain more to deepen your understanding or offer to meet the patient directly for a discussion. This can sometimes be reassuring for patients although it has the potential to be difficult for colleagues who have trained within a culture that is very different from the one that they ostensibly share with the patient. It also runs the risk of causing offence to the patient unless you offer this as a possibility rather than forcing it upon them (it may be that they would prefer not to see someone from this same cultural background as they hold very different personal beliefs).

■ **Don't forget child protection**. There may be instances when you feel uncomfortable about a certain part of the history or something doesn't seem quite right in the interaction between the child and the parents. It is important to consider the possibility of abuse if this happens, regardless of the cultural background of the family. It is dangerous to simply dismiss it as being 'a cultural difference'; share concerns with colleagues. All children are entitled to the same level of protection and safety regardless of their backgrounds and child abuse or neglect can never be justified on cultural or religious grounds. *For more information, see Chapter 4 – Child Protection and Safeguarding.*

Illiteracy

A recent UK government survey estimated that 5.1 million adults aged 16–65 years had literacy skills below the level required for completing normal functions such as paying household bills (Harding et al. 2011). Of this group, an estimated 2.4 million adults were functioning at or below a level which the report concluded would mean that they 'may not be able to describe a child's symptoms to a doctor'. This obviously impacts on providing care for children and the way in which we provide information to their parents. Providing written information seems like an obvious way to help parents to understand more about their child's condition but is not necessarily useful. Many adults will be too embarrassed to admit that they have difficulty with reading and writing. Try to get into the habit of routinely asking everyone in a matter-of-fact way if they have any difficulties with reading and writing. This can reduce your embarrassment about the topic and avoid you making assumptions about what parents can and can't do.

If a child is repeatedly missing their hospital appointments, might this be because their parents are unable to read the letter informing them of the time of the appointment?

Often patient information leaflets are translated into different languages to help families who do not speak English as their first language. However, they may not be literate in their own language either and therefore we should not assume that these leaflets are going to impart any useful information.

Here are some suggestions for finding out about literacy.

■ **Be straightforward about it**. Just as with any other potentially embarrassing topic, if the doctor is clearly embarrassed about asking the question then the parent or patient is going to be much more embarrassed about answering it.

■ **Make it routine**. If you ask everyone, it will become less daunting for you and you will become better at asking. It also avoids you making assumptions about certain families.

■ **Put it in context**. Explaining why you're asking the question can make it easier, for example saying something like 'We know that many adults in the UK have difficulties with reading and writing and a lot of the information we send from the hospital is in written form. Do you have any problems with reading or writing?'.

■ **Offer solutions**. If a parent does tell you that they have difficulty reading or writing, ask them what you or the hospital can do to improve the way that you communicate with them.

Consent

As mentioned many times above, it is important to include children as much as possible in decisions about their care. However, in most cases when working with young children, the child is not deemed competent to provide legal consent themselves and this must be given by their parents or carers on their behalf. An adult who is allowed to give consent on behalf of the child is referred to as having PARENTAL RESPONSIBILITY.

 Top Tip

Parental responsibility applies until the child is 18 years old in England, Wales and Northern Ireland or until 16 years old in Scotland. Many young people will be capable of providing their own consent to treatment before this age, as outlined in the text below.

Parental responsibility

All mothers automatically have PARENTAL RESPONSIBILITY for their own children (unless the child is legally adopted by someone else). The situation is more complicated when it comes to fathers and has changed within recent years.

In all parts of the UK, a father automatically has parental responsibility if he is married to the mother when the child is born or at the time of conception. Both parents keep parental responsibility if they later divorce.

An unmarried father can gain parental responsibility by:

■ making a Parental Responsibility Agreement with the child's mother

■ applying for a Parental Responsibility Order from the courts.

Unmarried fathers can also gain parental responsibility by jointly registering the birth with the mother and being named on the child's birth certificate as their father but this only applies to children born after:

■ 15th April 2002 in Northern Ireland

■ 1st December 2003 in England and Wales

■ 4th May 2006 in Scotland.

A stepparent (or the unmarried partner of a child's parent) can apply on their own to adopt the child, thus gaining parental responsibility. If an Adoption Order is granted to the stepparent then this cuts off the child's legal relationship with his or her 'absent' parent (the one who is not the partner of the new adoptive parent).

A doctor can treat a child without parental consent if:

■ it is an emergency

■ they have been given a court order to allow them to treat the child

■ the child is deemed to be capable of giving consent themselves (see At what age can children consent for themselves? section later in this chapter).

In most cases it is best to have parental consent if possible, but if the medical team cannot agree with the parents and the child is not capable of consenting for themselves then the doctors can apply for a court order to allow them to go ahead with treatment.

At what age can children consent for themselves?

There is no defined limit of age that determines whether or not a child is capable of giving consent and all must be assessed on a case-by-case basis. The important point to consider is whether or not the child has the capacity to consent to or refuse treatment. Capacity is not a concrete state of mind that means you either are or are not capable of giving consent; it refers to a person's ability to make a particular decision. Doctors can refer to criteria for 'GILLICK COMPETENCE' when deciding whether or not a child is capable of making a particular decision. For example, a child may have the capacity to consent to a simple treatment but lack the capacity to make a decision about a more complex procedure.

There are some slight differences in the default assumed position for children above and below the age of 16 and these are discussed in the following sections.

Children under sixteen years

Children who are under 16 years of age are presumed *not* to have capacity to consent as the default position. However, some children under 16 may be capable of consenting to treatment themselves. If this is the case then they are described as having 'GILLICK COMPETENCE'.

In order for a child to be deemed 'Gillick Competent' (and therefore legally able to consent to their own treatment) they must be able to:

■ understand what the treatment or procedure involves

■ weigh up the pros and cons of treatment and non-treatment

■ come to a reasoned decision.

GILLICK COMPETENCE is a generic term that applies to all children under 16 seeking medical treatment.

You may also hear people referring to the 'FRASER GUIDELINES'. Whilst these guidelines also deal with matters of consent in children under 16 years old, they apply only to decisions about giving contraceptive or abortion advice and treatment.

 Top Tip

Don't forget that children and young people are entitled to the same confidentiality as adults and information should usually only be shared with their consent. You can share information about a child or young person without their consent if they, or someone else, are at risk of death or serious harm. In these situations it may be best to discuss with the named doctor or nurse for child protection (without necessarily identifying the patient) to establish what information it may be necessary to share and with whom. Before you disclose any confidential information, you should inform the child or young person exactly what you will share, with whom and why this is necessary. *For more information on child protection, see Chapter 4 – Child Protection and Safeguarding.*

Sixteen and seventeen year olds

The law is slightly different for 16 and 17 year olds than for younger children. All children aged 16 and over are presumed to have the capacity to give consent to medical procedures unless proved otherwise. However, if someone of this age *refuses* consent for a treatment, the situation is much more complicated. It should certainly not be assumed that parents can override the young person's refusal by giving their consent. When a young person refuses treatment and the parents or doctors feel strongly that this is not in their best interests, you should try to find a resolution by spending time talking with the young person and their parents to establish the reasons for their differing views. Including other members of the multidisciplinary team can sometimes be helpful in this process and a resolution can often be found after negotiation and discussion. In rare circumstances when a solution cannot be agreed on, you should seek legal advice as you may need to apply through the courts for a decision about whether or not the young person should undergo treatment.

For more information about consent and confidentiality, see the General Medical Council guidance '0–18 years: guidance for all doctors', accessible at www.gmc-uk.org.

Useful websites

www.gosh.nhs.uk: the Great Ormond Street Hospital website is a fantastic resource with separate sections for children, teenagers and parents. It has lots of information about medical conditions and procedures, practical advice about staying in hospital and videos and stories of patients' experiences.

www.scope.org.uk: this charity provides support to disabled children and their families. It has lots of useful resources for professionals about communication with families and children.

www.thecommunicationtrust.org.uk: the Communication Trust is a collaboration of different organisations with expertise in speech, language and communication. It has lots of useful resources for professionals and parents on its website.

www.childbereavementuk.org: Child Bereavement UK runs courses on breaking bad news, providing support for families who have been bereaved or who have children with life-limiting conditions or complex needs. It also has lots of useful learning resources on its website and a support helpline for professionals and for family members.

www.bestbeginnings.co.uk: this website has a wealth of information (including lots of videos) for parents and professionals on a whole range of topics such as breastfeeding, parenting, premature and sick babies, and bereavement.

www.gmc-uk.org: the General Medical Council has copies of the guidance issued to doctors available on its website. It includes a publication specific to the management of children: '0–18 years: guidance for all doctors'.

Reference

Harding C, Romanou E, Williams J, et al. (2011) *2011 Skills for Life Survey: Headline Findings*. Department for Business, Innovation and Skills, London.

Mills K, Lalonde F, Clasen L et al. (2012) Developmental changes in the structure of the social brain in late childhood and adolescence. Soc Cogn Affect Neurosci, Oxford

Chapter 4
CHILD PROTECTION AND SAFEGUARDING

This is an upsetting and uncomfortable topic but sadly the abuse of children is much more commonplace than many of us probably imagine. A survey conducted by the NSPCC in 2011 found that over 25% of young adults reported experiencing severe abuse or neglect at some point during their childhood (Radford et al. 2011) Although some of these cases may represent short-term incidents, many children are subjected to abuse over a long period of time.

It can be difficult to understand how the very people who are supposed to be caring for the child are the ones causing them harm; it is important to acknowledge that sometimes you might feel upset or angered by the cases you see and try to find ways of dealing with this (see Chapter 10 – Looking After Yourself).

Child protection is of vital importance but is something that even the most experienced paediatricians find difficult to deal with at times. It can be a daunting prospect raising a concern that a child may be subject to abuse but remember that your discomfort with the topic is a symptom of how important it is and how much that child is suffering.

Different forms of abuse

Abuse can be categorised into several different types but they often do not occur in isolation (e.g. it is unlikely that a child subject to physical abuse has not suffered emotionally).

Physical abuse

See Box 4.1 for features suggestive of physical abuse in the history and examination.

This can be anything which causes physical harm to the child, such as hitting, shaking or biting, to scalding with boiling water or burning with cigarette ends. Fabricated or induced illness is also often categorised under physical abuse but for the purposes of this chapter is listed separately.

In the UK certain forms of physical punishment are still legal, despite this being in breach of the UN Convention of the Rights of the Child and calls from children's organisations for an outright ban (Bunting et al. 2008). This legal position has the potential to be confusing and difficult

The Hands-on Guide to Practical Paediatrics, First Edition. Rebecca Hewitson and Caroline Fertleman.
© 2014 John Wiley & Sons, Ltd. Published 2014 by John Wiley & Sons, Ltd.
Companion Website: www.wileyhandsonguides.com/paediatrics

Box 4.1   Clinical features suggestive of physical abuse

History

■ Delayed presentation (accident happened several days ago)

■ Story does not fit with the observed injuries. (Can you imagine what happened from the description you have been given? Does it sound likely or possible?)

■ Story inconsistent with the child's level of development

■ Vague account of events or unwitnessed injury (may also indicate neglect)

■ Different versions of story given by different people/at different times

■ Disclosure from the child

■ Unconcerned or aggressive parents

■ Repeated attendance to hospital or previous unusual injury

■ No story at all – parents who say 'I don't know, doctor, you tell me what happened'

Examination

■ Linear marks (e.g. from a belt or cane)

■ Bruising on buttocks, trunk, cheeks and ears all highly suspicious (accidental bruising normally on front and on bony prominences; shins, forehead, etc.)

■ *Any* bruise on an immobile child

■ Fractures:

– The younger the child, the more likely a fracture is secondary to abuse

– Most humeral fractures are suspicious of abuse (spiral fracture highly suspicious)

– Multiple fractures are much more common in abused children

– Rib fractures (particularly posterior) highly specific for abuse in very young children (Crawford et al. 2006)

■ Bite marks (human bites are in a U shape and rarely break the skin)

■ Retinal haemorrhages

■ Fingerprint bruises

■ Burns:

– Cigarette burns (deep, circular pits)

– Immersion scalds (glove or stocking distribution)

(Continued)

> — Bilateral burns and burns on face, feet and hands, legs and buttocks are commonly non-accidental
>
> — Accidental scalds tend to be in a 'splash' pattern over face and chest (for example, where a child has pulled a cup of hot coffee onto themselves) but may also be a cause for concern as they may reflect inappropriate supervision and indicate neglect

when knowing how to deal with cases. Here are some factors that may be helpful to consider.

■ **Who?** Physical punishment is illegal except if delivered by a parent, or someone acting on their behalf (e.g. grandparent).

■ **'Reasonable punishment'?** Parents can use 'mild' physical force to discipline a child if this is felt to be 'reasonable punishment', although in practice this defence is rarely used (Singleton 2010). What constitutes 'reasonable punishment' and at what point does a parent's actions become 'excessive'? Anything which leaves a mark on the skin or any hitting involving an implement certainly requires referral to social services. Other, 'milder' forms of punishment should be taken in a broader context and other factors about the parent–child interaction considered.

■ **Loss of control?** Many parents use physical punishment at times when they are feeling stressed or frustrated and feel out of control at the time and then immediately feel guilty afterwards (Bunting et al. 2008). It is important to be aware of this as use of physical punishment may be a sign that parents are not coping and need extra support.

 Top Tip

It is important to recognise that many things can stop people from raising concerns about abuse. Your own personal views on discipline of children can influence your decisions, as can fears of being culturally insensitive. Be aware of this and always have a low threshold for discussing with colleagues to gain a broader perspective.

Fabricated or induced illness (FII)

See Box 4.2 for clinical features suggestive of fabricated or induced illness.

This was previously also known as Munchausen syndrome by proxy and is often categorised under physical abuse. This type of abuse is very dangerous: research suggests that roughly 50% of children who have illness fabricated or induced experience long-term health problems as a result and 10% of these children die (Department for Children, Schools and Families 2008). It is most common in younger children (particularly the under-5s) but can occur in older children who may end up developing

It can be very difficult to distinguish between anxious parents responding to a child who has genuine symptoms and those who have grossly exaggerated, induced or fabricated symptoms in their child. A combination of the characteristics below can sometimes be suggestive of fabricated or induced illness.

- The clinical features do not make sense or fit with any diagnosis

- Symptoms only reported by carer (but never observed)

- Symptoms only occur when carers are present

- Carers intensively involved with children and don't allow anyone else to care for them

- Carers very involved with other families on the ward and hospital staff

- Carers don't appear to be appropriately concerned by abnormal results which may indicate serious illness in their child

- The most commonly presenting features in cases of fabricated or induced illness are fits and apparently life-threatening events (Davis et al. 2009)

- Feeding difficulties, reported allergies, poor growth

- Record of poor school attendance

- Extensive past medical history with investigation at multiple different hospitals

- Unexplained failure to respond to treatment

- As soon as one set of symptoms resolves, new ones are reported

- Impact on child's daily life (such as school attendance) far beyond what would be expected for a child with that diagnosis

- Carers inappropriately seeking opinions from multiple different doctors

abnormal illness behaviour themselves and colluding with their carers in fabricating or inducing illness in themselves.

■ **Fabricated illness** can range from exaggeration of symptoms to completely fictitious accounts of past medical history, altering hospital charts or producing fake letters or documents. Parents may also tamper with samples of bodily fluids in order to give false results (such as dripping blood into a child's urine sample). This fabrication of symptoms can result in the child missing a lot of school in order to attend hospital appointments. A lot of the harm caused comes from the medical profession as a result of the unnecessary and often unpleasant investigations the child has to undergo. In fact, the abuse can only continue with collusion from medical professionals; doctors can end up being complicit in the abuse.

Commonly reported symptoms are those that are difficult to verify without directly observing them, such as fits, vomiting, pain and frequency of passing urine.

Some children with fabricated or induced illness may have been totally well, whilst others may actually have an illness (either current or previous), the symptoms of which are being exaggerated or exacerbated by the parent's actions. Similarly, whilst some parents may be deliberately fabricating illness, others may genuinely believe that the child is unwell.

■ **Induced illness** is when the child's symptoms arise as a result of something the parent has done – for example, deliberate poisoning or suffocation, or, in a child who does actually need medication, giving the wrong dose deliberately or withholding the treatment altogether. This is extremely dangerous and must be acted upon immediately if suspected as the child's life can be in imminent danger.

 Top Tip

Do *not* discuss your suspicions with the parent or carer if you are considering the possibility of fabricated or induced illness. You need to discuss your concerns with a senior (preferably the named doctor or nurse for child protection) first so that decisions can be made about how to gather evidence (sometimes with the involvement of the police) and who will discuss the issue with the parents and when. Similarly, in rare instances when you suspect it is a member of staff who is responsible

for fabricating or inducing a child's illness, do not confront them directly but raise your concerns with a senior colleague. If, after discussion with a senior colleague, you feel that they have not adequately responded to your concerns then check your local child protection guidelines to find out who you should talk to next.

Emotional abuse

See Box 4.3 for clinical features suggestive of emotional abuse.

Emotional abuse can occur in isolation but is also an inevitable consequence of all forms of abuse of children. It is prolonged and pervasive behaviour which has a negative effect on a child's emotional development. Emotional abuse can involve:

■ being told that they are useless or not worthy of love

■ high criticism, low warmth

■ witnessing violence or aggression towards others (e.g. domestic violence)

■ unrealistic expectations of what a child can do at their age

■ overprotective and limiting of a child's normal social interactions and learning

■ being made to feel afraid or in danger

■ exploitation of children.

It can be one of the most difficult forms of abuse to detect and you may need information from many different people about the interactions they have observed between the parent and child (e.g. health visitors, school teachers, GP).

Box 4.3 Clinical features suggestive of emotional abuse

Children who have been subject to emotional abuse can present in many ways but often with emotional or behavioural problems. Observing the interactions between parent and child and also the way in which a parent talks about their child can provide useful information. Suggestive features in the parent–child interaction may be as follows.

■ Parent hardly talks to the child except when telling them to do something

■ Child appears anxious when parent is critical or verbally aggressive

■ Parent fails to respond to child's signals for help and does not appear concerned if the child is struggling with something

■ Parent offers little praise to the child

■ Parent does not play or interact with the child

The presenting features of a child who has been subject to emotional abuse can be very vague and vary between different age groups but can include the following.

Younger children
■ Language delay

■ FAILURE TO THRIVE

■ Sleep or feeding problems

■ Unconcerned by parent leaving them

■ Unable to play normally

School-age children
■ Poor school attendance and achievement

■ Angry, aggressive behaviour

■ Abnormal social interaction: this can range from an overly loud and 'attention-seeking' child who is inappropriately familiar with strangers, to a withdrawn and quiet child

■ Poor interactions with other children, few friends

■ Wetting and soiling

Adolescents
■ Depression, deliberate self-harm or eating disorders

■ Promiscuous or other risk-taking behaviour

■ Aggressive or antisocial behaviour

> **Box 4.4** Clinical features suggestive of neglect
>
> **History**
> ■ Persistent, severe infestations such as head lice or scabies
>
> ■ Explanation for injury suggests poor supervision (e.g. ingestion of harmful substance or young child playing outside late at night)
>
> ■ Frequent attendance to A&E with injury (suggests consistently poor supervision)
>
> ■ Repeated failure to attend for outpatient appointments
>
> ■ Child has not received immunisations
>
> ■ DEVELOPMENTAL DELAY or learning difficulties may suggest emotional neglect
>
> ■ Poor school attendance
>
> **Examination**
> ■ Smelly or very dirty child
>
> ■ Matted hair
>
> ■ Consistently wearing clothes inappropriate for the weather or the child's size
>
> ■ Evidence of malnutrition including FAILURE TO THRIVE
>
> ■ Dental caries

Neglect

See Box 4.4 for clinical features suggestive of neglect.

Neglect is a persistent failure of a parent to meet their child's basic emotional, psychological and/or physical needs. This can be deliberate or as a result of a parent's own difficulties such as mental illness. Disabled children and those with chronic illnesses are particularly vulnerable to neglect as their needs are often much greater.

Sexual abuse

See Box 4.5 for clinical features suggestive of sexual abuse.

Sexual abuse is difficult to detect and often is only discovered following disclosure from the child. Sexual abuse can include contact abuse or involving children in looking at or producing pornographic material or encouraging them to behave in sexually inappropriate ways.

> **Top Tip**
>
> Take any disclosure made by a child or a young person very seriously and bear in mind that often the abuse will have been happening for many years before a child has the courage to tell someone about it.

Box 4.5 Features suggestive of sexual abuse

There are many, non-specific physical symptoms which may occasionally be indicative of sexual abuse but have a broad medical differential diagnosis such as:

- vaginal bleeding in a prepubertal child
- recurrent vulvo vaginitis with or without dysuria
- rectal bleeding
- soiling or wetting in previously toilet-trained child (particularly soiling).

Certain behaviours may also point towards sexual abuse such as foreign body insertion into the anus or vagina, masturbation in public or a major unexplained change in the child's behaviour (anxiety, REGRESSION, poor school performance).

Certain 'sexualised' behaviours are normal in children of different ages and understanding these will help you to know when there is cause for concern. Sexualised behaviour in children is concerning if it is compulsive (i.e. you can't distract them or stop them from doing it), inappropriate for their stage of development or if it is affecting other areas of their life such as their school work or interaction with others. The following outline of *normal* sexual behaviour at different ages is adapted from an NSPCC factsheet (NSPCC 2010).

Preschool child (0–4 years)
- Is curious about other people's body parts
- Plays make-believe games mimicking families or visits to the doctor
- Talks about genitals
- Uses childish words for genitals (such as 'willy') freely
- Hugs and kisses others
- Touches their own genitals
- Shows their own genitals

Young child (5–9 years)
- Hugs and kisses others
- Is interested in other people's bodies
- Sometimes uses swear words or words relating to sex
- Plays make-believe games mimicking families or visits to the doctor
- May sometimes show their private body parts to others

(Continued)

- Touches own genitals
- May sometimes masturbate

Preadolescent (10–12 years)
- Is interested in other people's bodies
- May look at nude pictures, including on the internet
- Hugs and kisses others
- 'Dates' others their age
- Touches others' genitals
- Masturbates

Adolescent (13–16 years)
- Looks at nude pictures, including on the internet
- Masturbates privately
- Experiments sexually with others their own age
- Talks about sex with friends
- May use sexual language
- Asks questions about relationships and sexual behaviour

Physical signs
There are rarely any physical signs of abuse but there are a few things which are very concerning if found on examination.

- Bruises, particularly in the appearance of grip marks, over buttocks, thighs, lower abdomen and genitalia
- Any laceration or bruising around the penis
- Pregnancy
- Sexually transmitted infections

For details about specific management in cases of suspected sexual abuse, see the section below entitled 'What to do if you suspect child abuse'.

Teenage sexual behaviour
When dealing with teenagers, it can sometimes be difficult to know what constitutes normal teenage sexual behaviour and what is abusive or cause for concern. For more information on teenage sexual health see Chapter 8 – Teenagers. In the UK a child is not able to legally consent to any form of sexual activity until they are 16 years old. However, in some cases, for example sexual relations between two consenting 15 year olds, it may not be in the

best interests of these young people to pursue social services investigations and rarely would warrant police involvement. There are many things to consider when assessing whether or not the young person is at risk and what action would be in their best interests.

■ **How old is the patient?** For young people between the ages of 13 and 16, you must consider many things in your assessment of the case and should always involve your senior colleagues in the decision-making process. As a general rule, the younger the child, the more suspicious you should be that there is cause for concern. If the child is under the age of 13 then they are legally deemed incapable of consenting to sex and therefore all cases must be taken very seriously and referred to social services.

■ **Do you need to involve their parents?** Again this must be assessed on an individual basis. If a young person is deemed to be GILLICK COMPETENT then it may be possible to give them treatment with their consent without needing to consult or inform their parents (*for more information on Consent and Gillick Competence see Chapter 3 – Communication with Children and Their Parents*). It is always best to try to persuade the young person to involve their parents but you must try to respect their right to confidentiality if they are deemed capable of making informed decisions about their health.

■ **How old is the patient's sexual partner?** If the patient has a sexual partner who is much older than them then this should increase your level of

concern about the case. However, this is not to say that all relationships between young people of a similar age are not of concern. Violence and abuse within teenage relationships are also a problem and a high proportion of contact sexual abuse is perpetrated by people who are under 18 (Radford et al. 2011).

■ **Is there an imbalance of power in the relationship?** A large difference in age can contribute to this imbalance of power as can aggression, money and positions of authority. If someone is in a position of trust or authority (e.g. teacher, youth worker, nurse) then it is an offence for them to have sexual relations with a young person even if they are 16 or 17 years old.

■ **Was the child coerced, bribed or blackmailed into having sex with that person?** Did the child have sex with that person in return for money, food or accommodation? Were they threatened with what would happen to them if they told anyone? Consider if the child is at risk of or is being sexually exploited.

Maternal substance abuse in pregnancy

Another form of physical abuse is that of a pregnant woman causing damage to her unborn child. For example, if a pregnant women abuses heroin her baby is likely to have withdrawal symptoms after they are born as they have become physically dependent on opiates whilst *in utero*. This is known as neonatal abstinence syndrome and means that the baby may need to be

Box 4.6 Features that suggest a child is at risk of FEMALE GENITAL MUTILATION

■ Known previous FGM of other females in the family

■ Family of African, Middle or Far Eastern origin

■ Making preparations for the child to go on holiday

■ Absence from school or other normal activities

■ Arranging travel vaccinations

■ Child referring to a 'ceremony' or 'special procedure'

kept in hospital whilst being given regular oral morphine. The dose is gradually weaned down, a process which frequently takes several months to do.

Whilst the human fetus has no legal rights under English law, the moment that baby is born, they are entitled to exactly the same rights as all other children. In practical terms, this means that, if there are significant concerns regarding the unborn baby, child protection meetings are held and a plan put in place during the woman's pregnancy in anticipation of action which will be needed once that baby is born.

Female genital mutilation

See Box 4.6 for features suggesting a child is at risk of female genital mutilation.

FEMALE GENITAL MUTILATION (FGM) is a general term used for any process involving removal or injury of the external female genitalia for non-medical reasons. It can involve anything from cutting or piercing the genital area to total removal of the clitoris and labia minora or surgical narrowing of the vaginal opening.

Some key facts about FGM to be aware of include the following.

■ **There are no health benefits** associated with any of these procedures.

■ **FGM can cause significant harm** by causing severe pain, long-term fertility and childbirth problems, urinary retention and even result in death from bleeding or sepsis.

■ **FGM is recognised internationally as a violation of human rights** and there is a global strategy published by the World Health Organization to stop healthcare providers from performing FGM.

■ **It is illegal** in the UK both to perform FGM or to arrange for a girl to have FGM in another country (even if it is legal there).

■ **Involve your senior colleagues** and the child protection nurse or doctor immediately if you suspect that a girl is at risk of FGM.

Forced marriage and honour violence

See Box 4.7 for potential warning signs or indicators of possible forced marriage.

> **Box 4.7**   Risk factors or indicators suggesting forced marriage or honour violence
>
> ■ School absence
>
> ■ Decline in behaviour, performance or punctuality at school
>
> ■ Mental health problems: self-harm, eating disorders, depression, attempted suicide
>
> ■ Substance misuse
>
> ■ Siblings forced to marry
>
> ■ FEMALE GENITAL MUTILATION
>
> ■ Family disputes
>
> ■ Running away from home
>
> ■ Unreasonable restrictions set by parents

Forced marriage is when one or both of the potential spouses are under physical, psychological, emotional, sexual or financial pressure to marry. This is different from arranged marriages, in which families play an active role in finding a suitable partner but the decision rests with the two people potentially entering into the marriage about whether or not to go ahead. This can be associated with honour-based violence, which is physical assault, imprisonment or murder of a victim who is perceived to be bringing 'dishonour' or 'shame' on the family with their actions, or alleged behaviour.

■ Most victims of forced marriage are **females aged between 13 and 30 years**.

■ The majority of UK cases involve families of South Asian origin.

■ You normally only have one chance to help – **offer support immediately**.

■ Girls and women in forced marriages often experience **repeated violence and rape**.

What to do if you suspect that a child or young person may be at risk of forced marriage or honour-based violence

■ Do not use family members to translate.

■ See the child or young person alone (somewhere your conversation cannot be overheard).

■ Try questions like:

– How are things at home?

– Do you get on with your parents?

– Is your family supportive of what you want to do in life?

– What do your family want for you?

■ Immediately involve your seniors and the named child protection nurse or doctor.

■ Find a reason to keep the child or young person in the hospital or surgery whilst you find out more.

■ Contact the Forced Marriage Unit for advice (contact details available at http://www.gov.uk/forced-marriage).

For more information on forced marriage, including information leaflets, videos and practice guidelines for professionals, visit http:// www.gov.uk/forced-marriage.

Which children are most vulnerable to abuse?

It is important to avoid making assumptions about families and to be as objective as you can in your assessments. However, it is also important to be aware of certain risk factors which might make a child more likely to be subject to abuse and to be even more vigilant in considering these cases. The following characteristics of a child or their family make a child more likely to be subject to abuse. Many of them are interlinked.

■ **Disabled children**. They are more vulnerable to abuse because their needs are so much greater which can mean that parents or carers are unable to meet these or become stressed and vent their aggression on the child. Disabled children are often less able to communicate what has happened and therefore it can be much more difficult to detect which leaves them vulnerable to prolonged abuse.

■ **Premature babies**. Evidence suggests that children who were born prematurely are at greater risk of abuse. This may be because of interruption of normal bonding with parents whilst they are in a special care unit or because they often have greater needs with long-term health conditions and disabilities.

■ **Poverty**. Children from families with very little income are much more vulnerable to abuse.

■ **Parental substance misuse**. Parents who abuse drugs and alcohol are more likely to abuse their children. This can be because they act more impulsively and are in less control of their actions. Children can also be exploited by their parents in order to make money to continue to fuel their drug or alcohol habit.

■ **Mental health problems**. Adults who have mental health problems may be less able to cope with caring for their children.

■ **Domestic violence**. Witnessing domestic violence is child abuse in itself but children living in families where violence occurs are more likely to be subjected to physical abuse themselves. This may be when they try to step in to protect their mothers from abuse or a mother who is abused herself venting her frustration on her child.

■ **Under ones**. Babies who are less than 1 year old are at particular risk of serious abuse. They are eight times more likely than older children to be killed as a result of abuse (Cuthbert et al. 2011).

■ **Parental isolation**. Very young parents or single parents who lack support from their extended families may be more likely to be perpetrators of abuse.

■ **Dangerous dogs**. There is an association between owning dangerous dogs and child abuse. It is also worth considering the risk that the dog itself poses to the child as there are several reports of children having been killed by aggressive dogs.

What to do if you suspect child abuse

It is not just your moral duty to share concerns about child abuse; as a doctor you have professional obligations as outlined by the GMC (GMC 2012). This guidance applies to *all* doctors, even if your role involves looking after adults (as that adult may be a parent of a child at risk of abuse or pose a threat to the welfare of children). Child protection is everybody's business and training on the subject is compulsory for all doctors. You may also find it helpful to attend additional child protection courses such as those run by the Advanced Life Support Group (www.alsg.org).

 Top Tips

The most important rules in cases of suspected abuse

1 If you have any doubts or concerns, no matter how small, never ignore them

2 Tell someone senior

3 Ask the named doctor or nurse for child protection for advice

4 Document everything clearly and straight away

5 Take a detailed social history

6 Perform a full examination in good light

7 Follow your local child protection guidelines

This section details some general rules to follow when dealing with cases of suspected abuse. *For details about recognition and specific management of sexual abuse and child protection medicals. see the subsections below.*

If you suspect that a child may be subject to abuse, act as follows.

■ **Tell a senior colleague**. The crucial thing is to share your concerns with someone else, even if you feel that what you have noticed is relatively trivial or uncertain. You don't need to be able to give any kind of objective evidence at all to raise a concern with colleagues. If you feel uncomfortable and your gut instinct is that something is wrong, share this concern with others. Something which may seem pretty trivial when considered in isolation may become significant when combined with several different concerns that other professionals have had.

■ **Contact the named doctor or nurse**. By law, there must be a named doctor and named nurse for child protection at your hospital or in the community and they should be easily contactable (usually via bleep). Do not hesitate to get them involved; they will have a lot of experience and be able to help.

■ **Do not rely on someone else acting**. You could be the only person who has all the information to piece together and without your input the diagnosis may be missed.

■ **Document everything clearly and immediately**. Notes written in retrospect are much less useful as you may forget details. Document clearly and contemporaneously all of your history, including who you took the history from and who else was present. Use a BODY MAP to document all injuries and marks; again, do this at the time of examination rather than afterwards from memory. Record any conversations you have with other professionals about the case and any concerns you have raised. Your documentation may later be used as evidence in court so make sure that it would withstand the scrutiny of a lawyer; the quality of your notes could affect the outcome of a trial in cases of serious abuse.

■ **Consider sending the child for medical photographs**. It may be necessary to ask the medical photography team at your hospital to take photographs of marks or injuries as an objective record of their appearance. Photographs may also be taken by the police forensic team if they are involved.

■ **Take a particularly detailed social history**. This is always an important part of any paediatric clerking but should be even more detailed in cases of suspected abuse. Record the name of the child's school and the names and date of birth of their siblings. Ask if the family has had any involvement with social services and why. Ask if they currently have a named social worker. It is also useful to draw a family tree involving at least three generations (i.e. the child's grandparents), documenting where they live and if the child has much contact with them. This is useful as a way of checking how much support is available for the child's parents as social isolation of parents can be a risk factor for abuse. It is also necessary because in some cases the grandparents may have been abusing the child. You also need to ask about other people who live in the same house who may be distant relatives of the child or no relation at all, and if either of the child's parents has any children with different partners.

■ **Ask the child what happened**. Find an opportunity to ask the child about what happened, preferably without any of their relatives present. If the child does not speak English *do not use a family member to interpret* – contact a professional interpreter. *Do not use leading questions* such as 'Did mummy hit you?' as young children are easily manipulated and this may jeopardise a police investigation. Instead, try asking things like 'How did you get that mark on your arm?' and 'Have you got any other marks?'. Record the questions you ask the child and their responses to you verbatim. Police officers have guidance (ACHIEVING BEST EVIDENCE) on how to interview children to gather evidence so if you are in any doubt, it may be best to leave this to them.

■ **Check if the child is subject to a child protection plan**. Find out in which local authority the child lives and call them to ask if the family is known to them. If you are unsure, you can search using their postcode on the following website:

http://www.gov.uk/find-your-local-council. This can provide useful information about involvement of social services with the family and for what reasons.

■ **Do not be falsely reassured**. If you have a concern about potential child abuse, do not falsely reassure yourself and therefore fail to act. Just because a family has had no previous involvement with social services does not mean that you should drop your concerns as many cases of abuse go unreported for several years (Radford et al. 2011). Similarly, a seemingly loving interaction between parent and child does not exclude the possibility of abuse either from the parent or from someone else.

■ **Discuss with children's social care and/or the police**. After talking to your senior colleagues about the case, they may feel that an assessment by children's social services is needed. If there is an allegation or suspicion of a crime having been committed, you will also need to involve the police (although social care staff may make this decision on your behalf). Remember that it is the children's social care team which is responsible for co-ordinating and investigating safeguarding concerns so their involvement early on is crucial. *See below for more information about working with social services and the police.*

What should I say to the parents?

It is difficult to share concerns about abuse with parents and this may be best left to senior colleagues with more experience, but it is important for families to

 Top Tip

Do not inform parents if you suspect fabricated or induced illness, honour violence, forced marriage or FEMALE GENITAL MUTILATION as this can put the child in increased danger. In all cases, do not discuss with parents if to do so would place either yourself or the child in immediate danger.

know what to expect in terms of what will happen next so make sure that someone discusses this with them.

If you do have to raise this issue yourself, it may be helpful to say that it is your job to always consider the possibility that such injuries may have been caused intentionally and for that reason you are making a referral to social services so that they can help find out how and why this might have happened. You can let parents know that the Patient Advice and Liaison Services (PALS), which is a service available in most hospitals, is a good source of advice and support. The Children and Family Court Advisory and Support Service (CAFCASS) provides advice on its website for both parents and children and teenagers about court proceedings and what they involve (www.cafcass.gov.uk).

What to do if you suspect sexual abuse

In addition to the general principles outlined above, there are some specific management considerations when dealing with cases of suspected sexual abuse.

■ **Always involve the named nurse or doctor for child protection** in any cases of suspected sexual abuse as you are likely to need their expert input.

■ **Always inform your consultant** at the earliest possible opportunity so that they can help to manage the case.

■ **Do not ask leading questions** if a child makes an accusation of sexual abuse, as this can affect the reliability of any statements they make. Ask only open questions in order to find out more information and document verbatim your questions and the child's answers. If this is proving difficult and you are not getting the information you need then get someone senior involved as it may be more appropriate for the child to be questioned by a police officer who has been trained in questioning children for providing evidence.

■ **Contact children's social care** immediately as they will be able to advise on the appropriate next steps and co-ordinate involvement of other services such as the police, community paediatricians or acute sexual assault specialist centres if necessary. You may wish to involve the police immediately by calling them yourself in cases of alledged recent rape or sexual assault, but make sure that you agree a clear plan with children's social care about who will contact the police and how urgently their involvement is needed.

■ **Gain consent from the child and parents for any examination**, although it may be more appropriate to leave intimate examinations to an experienced colleague such as those in specialist sexual assault centres or community paediatricians.

■ **Take a chaperone with you when examining the child**.

■ **Use the chain of evidence process if collecting any samples**. If the child has been acutely sexually assaulted then it may be possible to collect forensic evidence. In most cases this is still possible up to 7 days after the assault occurred, but evidence is best obtained as quickly as possible, preferably within 24 h of the assault. Some of this evidence can be collected by police using the 'early evidence kit' (for example, to collect urine and mouth swabs) and the child will then need to be referred urgently to see a doctor who specialises in sexual assault. If you are planning to take any swabs (e.g. for detection of sexually transmitted diseases) then this must be done using the CHAIN OF EVIDENCE process. This involves the person who collects the samples filling in a chain of evidence form with their own details, signature and date and all the child's details. After this, any other person who handles the sample (including any porters who carry the sample to the laboratory) must sign and date the same form. This is so that, if the result of the swab is subsequently used in court as evidence of abuse, it can be proved that this was definitely the right result for the right patient and has not been tampered with. Examples of CHAIN OF EVIDENCE forms can be found in the appendices of the RCPCH *Child Protection Companion* (Crawford et al. 2006). In practice, it may sometimes be better to leave all swabs to be done at the specialist centre to avoid undue distress for the child or teenager from repeated examinations.

■ Refer urgently to a specialist centre in cases of acute assault. As mentioned above, this should normally be co-ordinated by children's social care who will be aware of local processes. However, if you wish to find out where the local rape and sexual assault referral centre for your hospital or GP practice is, you can go to the NHS Choices website and search under the 'health services near you' tab (http:// www.nhs.uk/service-search). This will find local services including contact details. Not all centres will provide services for children so it is best to call them to find out or to ask the advice of the social worker.

Child protection medicals

Part of the child protection process normally involves a specialist assessment by a community paediatrician. These are often referred to as 'child protection medicals' and involve a detailed assessment of the child involving a thorough history and top-to-toe examination with full documentation of all findings. As a junior doctor, you may have the opportunity to work as part of a community paediatric team but will always be supervised by a registrar and a consultant.

Some key points about child protection medicals include the following.

■ Use the dedicated proforma if available. Many community clinics will have proformas for use in child protection medicals. This can be a helpful prompt for specific questions and often contains BODY MAPS for documenting your examination findings.

■ Obtain written consent. Ask the person with PARENTAL RESPONSIBILITY who is accompanying the child to sign to give their consent for the medical (bearing in mind that this may be the social worker in some cases).

■ Write a summary report. In order to make your assessment useful for others, write a short report of your key history and examination findings and your conclusions about the allegation (e.g. your opinion about whether or not your findings were consistent with accidental or deliberate injury).

■ Discuss all cases with your consultant, ask them to read your final report and check that they are happy with your proposed management plan.

■ Communicate your report findings to social care. This is a crucial part of the process – there is no point doing a detailed assessment if you do not share this information to allow social workers to decide about the necessary next steps.

Working with social care, education and the police

See Figures 4.1, 4.2, 4.3 and 4.4 for an overview of the child protection process.

Having a basic knowledge of the roles and responsibilities of different agencies and the formal processes surrounding child protection cases is crucial for understanding where you fit into the whole process as a doctor.

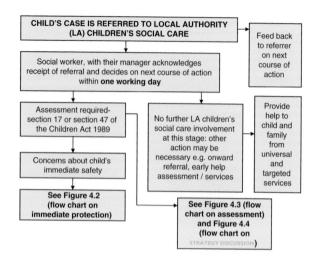

```
┌─────────────────────────────────────────────┐      ┌──────────────┐
│   CHILD'S CASE IS REFERRED TO LOCAL AUTHORITY │─────▶│  Feed back   │
│        (LA) CHILDREN'S SOCIAL CARE            │      │  to referrer │
└─────────────────────────────────────────────┘      │  on next     │
                     │                                │  course of   │
                     ▼                                │  action      │
┌─────────────────────────────────────────────┐      └──────────────┘
│   Social worker, with their manager acknowledges │
│ receipt of referral and decides on next course of │
│        action within one working day           │
└─────────────────────────────────────────────┘
```

Assessment required-
section 17 or section 47 of
the Children Act 1989

No further LA children's
social care involvement
at this stage: other
action may be
necessary e.g. onward
referral, early help
assessment / services

Provide
help to
child and
family
from
universal
and
targeted
services

Concerns about child's
immediate safety

**See Figure 4.2
(flow chart on
immediate protection)**

**See Figure 4.3 (flow
chart on assessment)
and Figure 4.4
(flow chart on
STRATEGY DISCUSSION)**

Figure 4.1 Action taken when a child is referred to local authority children's social care services. Reproduced from Department of Education (2013) Working Together to Safeguard Children, under Crown copyright licence.

There is national guidance on child protection called *Working Together to Safeguard Children* which outlines the responsibilities of different organisations and individuals. This document is available online at http:// www.education.gov.uk/aboutdfe/statutory National guidance on child protection changes quite frequently so the following section is a rough overview only; always check with your local named doctor or nurse for child protection and refer to local guidelines for the most up-to-date information.

Social care

Children's social care are responsible for co-ordinating any child protection proceedings and ensuring the safety and well-being of children living within the local authority area. You can call children's social care for advice if you have concerns about a child's welfare or want to know if they have had any previous involvement with the family. It is important to make prompt referrals to social services in order to prevent problems from escalating and ensure that the child remains safe. Making a good initial referral to social care is vital to ensuring that the case is managed promptly. *See Box 4.8 for how to make a good referral to social services.*

Police

If you suspect that a crime has been committed (for example, in cases of assault or sexual abuse) then the police

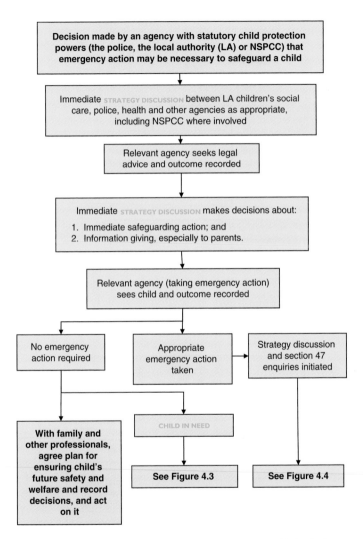

Figure 4.2 *Immediate protection. Reproduced from Department of Education (2013)* Working Together to Safeguard Children, *under Crown copyright licence.*

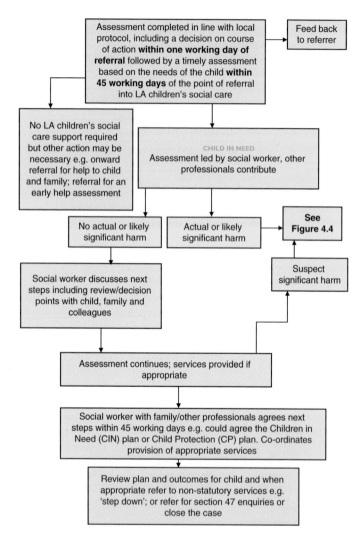

Figure 4.3 Action taken for an assessment of a child under the Children Act 1989. Reproduced from Department of Education (2013) Working Together to Safeguard Children, under Crown copyright licence.

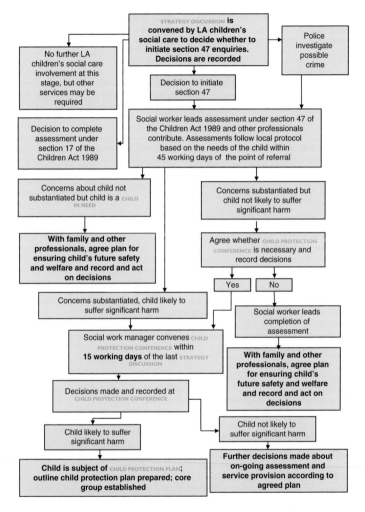

Figure 4.4 Action following a strategy discussion. Reproduced from Department of Education (2013) Working Together to Safeguard Children, *under Crown copyright licence.*

will also need to be involved. This is usually done by the social worker following your referral to them, but clarify this with them. Each police service will have a dedicated child abuse investigation team (CAIT). They will have an early evidence kit to allow prompt collection of evidence from skin swabs. Keeping the child's clothes is also really important as evidence can remain on clothes for a very long period of time and may be crucial to a criminal prosecution.

The processes involved in child protection cases can seem complex and doctors are not always aware of their

---

Box 4.8 How to make a referral to children's social services

Making a good referral to children's social services is crucial to allow them to assess how quickly they need to see the family and if emergency intervention is required. Each local authority will have its own process for referrals to social services which should be outlined in your hospital's child protection policy. If unsure, you can check with the named child protection nurse or doctor to ensure that you follow the correct referral procedure. There are, however, some general rules to follow.

Check which local authority to refer to

This is determined by the child's home address and can vary by street in some big cities. You can search for a patient's local authority using their address at http:// www.gov.uk/find-your-local-council.

Call the relevant local authority to discuss the case with a social worker

In many cases you will be put through to an administrative member of staff who is receiving the calls and will take down basic details including your contact number so that a social worker can call you back to discuss the case. Make sure that you have all the relevant information to hand so that you don't waste their time and can give a clear account of the case and what your concerns are. It may help you to fill in the written referral form before making the phone call to order your thoughts and make sure that you know all the relevant information.

Make a written referral

You are obliged to follow up any referral over the phone with a written referral. Legally you must do this within 48 h but ideally, you should try to do it the same day. The information that you provide in your referral will allow a social worker to decide how urgently they need to see the child and their family so make sure that you fill in as much detail as possible, including specific examples of what has caused you to be concerned and any relevant information about

---

the child's level of development. Remember that social workers are not medically trained so avoid using medical jargon or abbreviations.

Document what you have done
Make sure that you record the outcome of the telephone conversation in the child's notes and file a copy of your written referral in the notes too along with documentation of where you sent the referral to and when (fax, e-mail, etc.). Be aware that if your local system involves emailing a referral, this must be done using your NHS account in order to ensure that the information is secure.

Provide a contact number
Once the social worker has made a decision about the case, they will contact the person who made the referral to let them know within one working day. It can be sensible to provide a bleep number which is held 24/7 (such as an on-call bleep) so that the message will be received regardless of whether or not you are at the hospital. If you know that you are not going to be on duty, make sure that you hand over details of the case to the person who will be carrying the bleep so that they can have a useful conversation with the social worker about what is planned for that child.

role within these. The questions below address some of the processes involved and jargon used in child protection cases.

I've made a referral to social services; what happens next?

Within one working day of you sending your referral, a social worker should contact you to let you know what needs to be done next. If you don't hear from them, make sure that you chase it up and that the referral has not been missed.

On the basis of your written referral, the social worker will decide either that no further input is needed from social services or that they need to complete an assessment of the child and their family. If they decide that a child needs further assessment then they will also decide how

urgently this needs to happen and if any immediate action is needed to keep the child safe.

What if you are worried about the immediate safety of the child?

Social services, the police and the National Society for the Prevention of Cruelty to Children (NSPCC) all have powers to act in an emergency if there is a risk to the child's life or they are at risk of serious immediate harm. If parents are co-operating then it may be safest to keep the child in the hospital for a short period of time whilst an immediate STRATEGY DISCUSSION takes place. If the child is at home or parents leave the hospital with the child then the local authority can apply through

the courts for an EMERGENCY PROTEC-
TION ORDER (EPO) which gives them
the authority to remove a child from
their home.

What is a section 17 investigation?

If, on the basis of your referral, a social
worker decides that further assessment
is needed then this is authorised legally
by section 17 of the Children Act 1989.
This is sometimes referred to as an
INITIAL ASSESSMENT. The social worker
will contact the various different agencies (education, police, etc.) to gather
information about the child's social circumstances and may also contact you to
find out more detail about their medical
history. They will also conduct interviews
with the child and their family. After they
have completed their assessment, they
will make a decision about whether or
not that child is a CHILD IN NEED.

Who is a child in need?

This is defined by the Children Act of
1989 as any child who will need input
from services in order to reach or maintain a good standard of health and
development. This means that all children with disabilities and 'LOOKED-AFTER
CHILDREN' are automatically defined as
being a CHILD IN NEED. This also includes
children who are at risk of significant
harm as a result of abuse or neglect.

Who is a looked-after child?

A LOOKED-AFTER CHILD is one for whom
the local authority is responsible. This
normally means that the local authority
shares PARENTAL RESPONSIBILITY with
the child's parents and that the local
authority is responsible for finding a
suitable place for the child to live (usually, with a suitable relative, in a care
home or with a foster family).

What happens after it is decided that a child is in need?

If the child has not come to significant
harm and this is not likely then the
social worker will discuss with the family and the child what further support
they might need and co-ordinate the
provision of those services. If the child
has suffered, or is likely to suffer, significant harm then the social worker will
arrange a STRATEGY DISCUSSION.

What is a strategy discussion?

This is also sometimes known as a
STRATEGY MEETING. This can be in the
form of a meeting or can be done with
separate phone calls to each of the
agencies. As a minimum, it must involve a
social worker and their manager, a police
officer and a health professional but may
include other relevant people such as
the person who made the referral and
teachers from the child's school or nursery. This is used as a way of everyone
sharing relevant information which
allows decisions to be made on whether
any immediate action is needed to keep
the child safe, whether an enquiry
should take place under section 47 of
the Children Act, and if and when any
criminal investigation will take place.

What is a section 47 enquiry?

This is sometimes referred to as a CORE ASSESSMENT. This is a detailed assessment led by social services and involves them finding out more about the child's needs and their parents' ability to meet these needs. It involves working with police, health and education to gather information and interviews with parents and the child. Health professionals may be asked to carry out more detailed assessments of the child's development. The social worker then makes a decision about whether or not to convene a CHILD PROTECTION CONFERENCE.

What is a child protection conference?

This is a formal meeting involving family members (including the child if appropriate), with any relevant supporters, advocates or professionals who have been involved with the child or the family. Expert advice may be needed from orthopaedic doctors, plastic surgeons specialising in burns or paediatric radiologists when thinking about mechanism of injury. The purpose of the meeting is to decide if the child is at risk of significant harm in the future and therefore should be subject to a CHILD PROTECTION PLAN.

What is a child protection plan?

This is a plan which outlines what needs to be done and by whom in order to keep the child safe. The type of abuse to which the child was being subjected is recorded as part of the plan (i.e. physical, sexual, etc.) and a lead social worker will be allocated to be in charge of the case and ensure that all the plans are implemented.

What is a child protection review conference?

Three months after a CHILD PROTECTION PLAN is put in place, a review conference is held to see if any changes to the plan are needed or if a protection plan is no longer necessary. If the child remains subject to a child protection plan then this continues to be reviewed at a child protection review conference every 6 months.

What is the child protection register?

The child protection register used to be a list kept by the local authority of all children who were felt to be at risk of significant abuse. You may still hear people referring to the child protection register but there is now just a record of children who are subject to a CHILD PROTECTION PLAN.

What stops us from considering the possibility of abuse?

There are many barriers which can stop us from considering the possibility of abuse or from raising our concerns with other people. Having an awareness of these barriers may help you to recognise and overcome some of them.

■ **We don't want to miss a treatable disease**. What if the bruising is because of a rare bleeding disorder? No-one wants to miss a medical pathology but consideration of abuse in your differential diagnosis should happen *at the same time* as investigations for organic pathology.

■ **We like to think the best of people**.

■ **We are afraid of how parents will react to the diagnosis** and dread having to have an uncomfortable conversation with them when raising the possibility of abuse.

■ **We are afraid of what will happen if we are wrong**. What if there is a medical explanation for the injuries but the parents have been arrested and taken away from their child?

■ **We fear being ridiculed by colleagues for 'overreacting'**.

■ **We think that the relationship between the child and parent is a very loving one** and therefore couldn't possibly be abusive. This is a common mistake and often falsely reassures people. Most abusive parents do love their children but don't have the right parenting skills or mechanisms for coping with their own frustration or anger.

■ **Our default mode of operation in medicine is to believe what the patient or parent is telling us**.

■ **Sometimes the possibilities are too horrid and we prefer not to believe them to be true**.

■ **We don't listen carefully enough to what children and young people are telling us**.

■ **We know the family well**.

■ **Cultural differences**. We don't want to be accused of being racist or ignorant of cultural practices. However, regardless of a child's cultural or religious background, they should be entitled to the same level of protection and child abuse or neglect can never be justified on religious or cultural grounds.

■ **Previous referral to social services was rejected**. If the last time you referred a child to the children's social service team, they were not concerned and have not investigated further then this could make you more reluctant to send another referral. Remember that it is far better to have a low threshold for asking for advice than to miss a serious case.

■ **We fear the high-profile nature of some child protection cases**. There have been several very high-profile cases of child abuse in recent years which have had serious consequences for the doctors involved. We fear being the ones to miss a serious case but this is weighed against the risk of accusing someone wrongly of abusing a child and becoming scrutinised yourself. The idea of being pulled up in front of the General Medical Council or featuring in the news fills all of us with fear.

Useful websites

NSPCC: www.nspcc.org.uk has loads of information for parents, professionals and children about abuse and keeping safe.

Children and Family Court Advisory and Support Service (CAFCASS): www.cafcass.gov.uk has information for families and children who are going through court proceedings.

www.rapecrisis.org.uk: charity to support women and girls who have been subject to sexual violence.

NHS Choices: www.nhs.uk. The 'services near you' section of the website allows you to search for rape and sexual assault referral centres in your area.

Forced Marriage Unit: http:// www.gov.uk/ forced-marriage. Contains useful informa-tion, videos and advice for both profes-sionals and patients.

References

Bunting L, Webb MA, Healy J (2008) *The 'smacking Debate' in Northern Ireland – Messages from Research*. NSPCC, Northern Ireland.

Crawford M, Ghulam S, Herbison J, et al. (2006) *Child Protection Companion*. Royal College of Paediatrics and Child Health, London.

Cuthbert C, Rayns G, Stanley K (2011) *All babies Count: Prevention and Protection for Vulnerable Babies*. NSPCC, London.

Davis P, Glaser D, Humphrey C, et al. (2009) *Fabricated or Induced Illness by Carers (FII): A Practical Guide for Paediatricians*. Royal College of Paediatrics and Child Health, London.

Department for Children, Schools and Families (2008) *Safeguarding Children in Whom Illness is Fabricated or Induced*. DCSF Publications, Nottingham.

General Medical Coucnil (2012) *Protecting Children and Young People: The Responsibilities of All Doctors*. General Medical Council, Manchester.

NSPCC (2010) *Sexual Behaviour of Children: What is Normal, Worrying or Abusive?* NSPCC, London.

Radford L, Corral S, Bradley C, et al. (2011) *Child Abuse and Neglect in the UK Today* NSPCC, London.

Singleton R (2010) *Physical Punishment: Improving Consistency and Protection*. Department for Children, Schools and Families, London.

Chapter 5
COMMON PAEDIATRIC EMERGENCIES

With all emergencies remember to **get help early**. Put out a paediatric crash call or call the emergency services to get help quickly (in the UK dial 2222 in any hospital or 999 in the community) if a child is acutely unwell; do not wait until they are peri-arrest.

Basic Life Support

See Fig. 5.1 for Basic Life Support algorithm. See Video 1 for how to perform paediatric Basic Life Support.

There are some differences from adult Basic Life Support because of children's smaller size and also because in children cardiorespiratory arrest is usually secondary to hypoxia, whereas in adults there is often a cardiac cause. For this reason, the pattern starts with rescue breaths rather than chest compressions.

An easy way to remember the steps needed for Basic Life Support is with the pneumonic DRS ABC.

Danger

First of all check that it is safe for you to approach the child, particularly if in a community setting and you are a first responder. Put on gloves and apron if available.

Response

Stimulate the child to establish whether they are responsive. You can do this by loudly calling the child's name or saying 'are you all right?'. Never shake a baby or child to check for a response in case they have a cervical spine injury. You can gently move their arm to try to get a response whilst holding their head still.

Shout for help

If the child is unresponsive shout for help but do not leave the child. If someone comes to help you, ask them to dial 2222 in hospital or 999 in the community. In hospital, ask the person to put out a paediatric arrest call or in the community ask the person to tell the ambulance service that the child is unconscious. Ask them to come back to help once they have made the phone call. If no-one comes to help you do not delay but move straight to giving Basic Life Support.

The Hands-on Guide to Practical Paediatrics, First Edition. Rebecca Hewitson and Caroline Fertleman.
© 2014 John Wiley & Sons, Ltd. Published 2014 by John Wiley & Sons, Ltd.
Companion Website: www.wileyhandsonguides.com/paediatrics

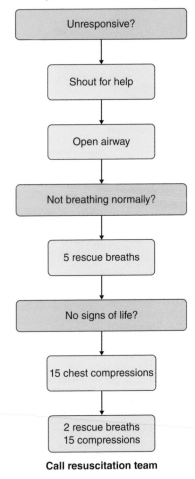

Paediatric basic life support
(Healthcare professionals with a duty to respond)

Unresponsive?

Shout for help

Open airway

Not breathing normally?

5 rescue breaths

No signs of life?

15 chest compressions

2 rescue breaths
15 compressions

Call resuscitation team

Figure 5.1 Paediatric Basic Life Support algorithm. Reproduced with permission from Resuscitation Council UK.

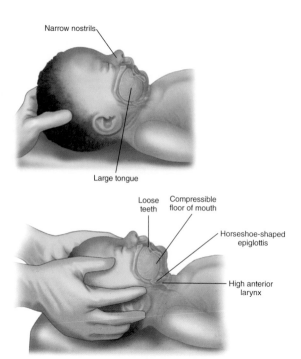

Figure 5.2 *Opening the airway of an infant using a head tilt and chin lift. (a) Airway occluded. (b) Airway opened using head tilt and chin lift.*

Airway

■ **Look in the mouth**. If you can see anything obvious occluding airway then remove it if it is easy to do so but don't sweep with your finger further than you can see as you may end up pushing something further down into the airway.

■ **Open the airway**. Use either a 'head tilt, chin lift' or 'jaw thrust' manoeuvre. Always use a jaw thrust if you suspect a cervical spine injury.

– **Head tilt, chin lift**. Put one hand on the forehead and one finger under the bony part of the jaw and tilt the head. For babies up to 1 year old, move their head so that it is in a neutral position (i.e. with their face parallel to the surface they are lying on). For children, their head should be moved so that their neck is partly extended into a 'sniffing' position. Be careful to place your fingers on the bony part of the jaw as pressing on the soft tissues can occlude the airway. See Fig. 5.2 for

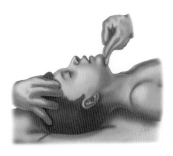

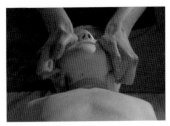

Figure 5.4 Jaw thrust manoeuvre.

Figure 5.3 Opening the airway of a child using head tilt and chin lift.

babies and Fig. 5.3 for child head position in head tilt, chin lift.

– Jaw thrust. Position yourself above the child's head so that you are looking down towards their feet. Place the ring and middle finger of each hand at the angle of the jaw on both sides and the fleshy part of your thumb on their cheekbones. Using both hands together, pull up on the angle of the jaw with your fingers and press down with your thumbs in order to bring the lower jaw forward. *See Fig. 5.4.*

Breathing

Once you have opened the airway you need to assess for normal breathing.

■ **Look, listen and feel**. Look for chest and abdominal movements, listen for airflow at mouth and nose and feel for breath on your cheek. This should be done for no more than 10 sec.

■ **Give five rescue breaths**. If the child is not breathing or is taking only occasional gasps then give five rescue

breaths. If you don't have access to any equipment then seal your lips tightly around the child's mouth and pinch their nose, or for a baby seal your lips around their nose and mouth. If you have a pocket mask you can use this to deliver rescue breaths using your breath. If you have access to a bag-valve mask this can be used to deliver the breaths.

■ **Watch for chest movement**. If there is no chest movement as you deliver a rescue breath, reposition the child's head to ensure that the airway is open and make sure that you have a tight seal around the child's nose and mouth before delivery of the next breath.

Circulation

■ **Feel for a pulse and look for signs of life**. After you have delivered the five rescue breaths, feel briefly for a pulse and look for signs of life. *This should take no more than 10 sec.* In a child, feel for carotid or femoral pulses; in an infant, feel for brachial or femoral pulses. It can be difficult to be sure of whether or not you can feel a pulse within 10 sec so also look for signs of life, which might be coughing or gagging in response to rescue breaths or movement.

■ **Start chest compressions**. If there are no signs of life or the child's pulse is not palpable or their heart rate is less then 60 beats per minute, commence chest compressions. If you are in any doubt about whether or not you can feel a pulse and the child is showing no signs of life, commence chest compressions.

– **Where?** In a child, feel for the xiphisternum and place the heel of your hand just above this point (on the lower half of the sternum). You can use two hands if needed. In babies, feel for the xiphisternum and place two fingers just above this point (on the lower half of the sternum). If there are two of you providing Basic Life Support then a more effective method is for one person to stabilise the airway whilst the other wraps their hands around the baby's chest and uses both thumbs to compress at this point on the lower half of the sternum. See Fig. 5.5 for two-hand technique.

– **How hard?** Don't be afraid to press quite hard. The chest compressions need to compress to a depth of at least a third of the chest in order to be effective.

– **How fast?** Chest compressions should be given at a rate of 100–120 beats per minute.

– **How many?** Do 15 chest compressions.

– **What next?** After your 15 chest compressions, give two more breaths and continue at a ratio of 15:2.

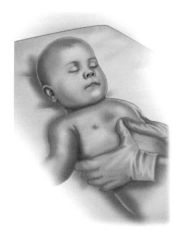

Figure 5.5 Two-hand technique for giving chest compressions in babies.

Continue like this until the child moves or takes a breath. *After 1 min of resuscitation if no-one has come to help, go and call the emergency services (999) yourself or put out a paediatric crash call if you are in hospital (2222).* As soon as you have done this, restart chest compressions and ventilations until help arrives.

Choking child

See Fig. 5.6 for paediatric choking management algorithm. See Video 1 for a demonstration of how to manage a choking child.

Choking often occurs when children are playing or eating and is frequently witnessed by their parents or carers who will give a clear history

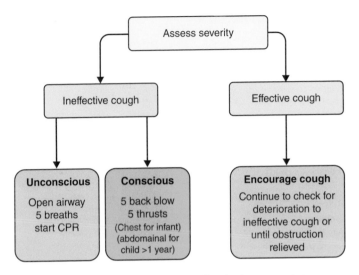

Figure 5.6 Paediatric choking management algorithm. CPR, cardiopulmonary resuscitation. Reproduced with permission from Resuscitation Council UK.

of the child putting something in their mouth and then choking.

History

Ask about:

■ sudden onset

■ playing with small objects just prior to onset

■ eating

■ coughing.

Symptoms

■ Panic

■ Coughing

■ Unable to breathe

Signs

■ Stridor

■ Gagging

■ Coughing

■ Cyanosis

■ Decreased consciousness

Immediate management

Is the child coughing effectively or not?

■ **Effective coughing**. This means that they are able to talk or cry, make a loud sound whilst coughing and are able to take a deep breath before each cough. If the child is coughing effectively simply reassure them and encourage them to continue coughing.

■ **Ineffective coughing**. The child has a silent or quiet cough and is unable to vocalise or breathe. They may have cyanosis or reduced conscious level. If this is the case then what you do depends on whether or not the child is conscious.

Managing ineffective coughing (conscious child)

■ Shout for help.

■ Give five back blows.

− **Child**. Deliver short, sharp blows between the shoulder blades with the heel of your hand. The aim should be to relieve the obstruction with each blow rather than to deliver all five.

− **Baby**. Sit on a chair or kneel on the floor. Support the baby's head by placing your thumb and index finger around the lower jaw, taking care not to compress the soft tissues under the jaw. Place the baby face down across your lap and deliver five sharp blows to the middle of the back with the heel of the hand. Do not be afraid to do this quite forcefully in order to relieve the obstruction. See *Fig. 5.7 for how to hold a baby for back slaps.*

■ **Deliver five abdominal or chest thrusts**. If the back blows do not relieve the airway obstruction, deliver five abdominal thrusts.

− **Child**. Stand behind the child, clench one of your fists and place it against the child's abdomen approximately midway between the umbilicus and xiphisternum. In small children you may

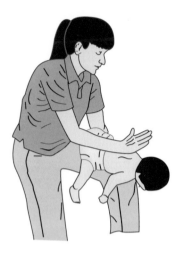

Figure 5.7 How to hold a baby to deliver back slaps if they are choking.

need to kneel down or stand the child on a chair in order to do this effectively. Pull sharply inwards and upwards five times. See *Fig. 5.8 for how to perform abdominal thrusts on a child.*

− **Baby**. Turn the baby over on your knee, keeping them in a head-down position. Place two fingers just above the xiphisternum (in the same site as for chest compressions) and press down with short, sharp thrusts. These should be slower and more forceful than for chest compressions. The aim is to remove the obstruction with each thrust rather than to deliver all five and these need to be done firmly to generate enough intrathoracic pressure to relieve the obstruction. See *Fig. 5.9 for how to hold a baby for chest thrusts.*

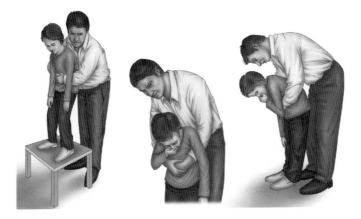

Figure 5.8 How to perform abdominal thrusts on a child if they are choking.

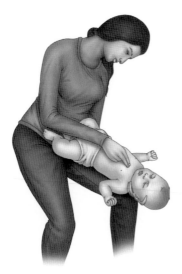

Figure 5.9 How to hold a baby to deliver chest thrusts if they are choking.

Managing ineffective coughing (unconscious child)

If a child or baby becomes unconscious as a result of choking, commence Basic Life Support as detailed above. Recheck the mouth after each cycle of chest compressions to look for a foreign body that may have been dislodged.

Advanced Life Support

See Fig. 5.10 for a paediatric Advanced Life Support algorithm.

If you are in a hospital setting you will have access to more equipment which will allow you to perform more advanced support to children who are unresponsive. Follow the same steps as for Basic Life Support but you can use equipment to aid the process.

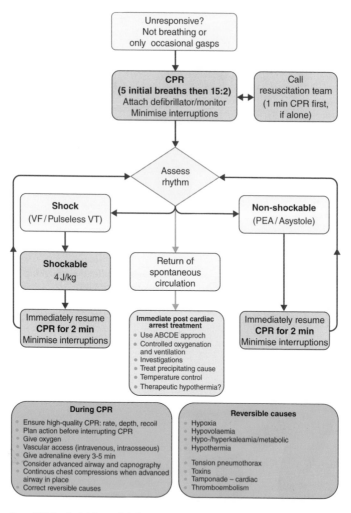

Figure 5.10 Paediatric Advanced Life Support algorithm. CPR, cardiopulmonary resuscitation. PEA, pulseless electrical activity; VF, ventricular fibrillation; VT, ventricular tachycardia. Reproduced with permission from Resuscitation Council UK.

Airway management

■ **Airway manoeuvres**. Use a 'head tilt, chin lift' or a 'jaw thrust' as detailed in the Basic Life Support section. *For examples of how to do each of these manoeuvres see Video 1.*

■ **Airway adjuncts**. If you are struggling to keep the child's airway open using the manoeuvres mentioned above, you can use pieces of equipment to help keep the airway open.

– **Oropharyngeal (Guedel) airway**. You can use one of these to help keep the tongue and soft tissues from occluding the airway but they will only be tolerated in a child who is unconscious. If the child's gag reflex is intact, insertion of a GUEDEL may induce vomiting and it should be removed. Check you are using the correct size by making sure that the airway is long enough to reach from the middle of the incisors to the angle of the jaw when resting along the side of the child's face. It can help to use a tongue depressor as you insert it to get the airway in the correct position.

– **Nasopharyngeal airway**. In a child with facial injury or lip and tongue swelling or a child who is having a seizure, this can be a useful type of airway adjunct. It is sometimes also better tolerated than oropharyngeal airways in children who are not completely unconscious. Use of a nasopharyngeal airway is contraindicated in trauma patients with a suspected base of skull fracture. Make sure that you put a safety pin through the end of the tube which is to remain outside the child if you are not using a brand of tube that has its own stopper on the end. This is to prevent the airway from accidently sliding all the way into the nasopharynx. The correct airway size to use is one that is roughly the same diameter as the child's little finger. If a small size of nasopharyngeal airway is not available a shortened endotracheal tube may be used.

■ **Tracheal intubation**. The above measures are usually only temporary solutions to open the airway and a child who remains unconscious despite initial resuscitation is likely to need tracheal intubation. This should only be done by someone experienced so do not attempt this on your own unless you have had adequate training.

Breathing management

If a child is not breathing or is only making occasional gasping breaths then start Basic Life Support. If you are in a hospital setting you may have access to the following equipment to help you with this.

■ **Pocket masks**. These are facemasks designed for giving mouth-to-mouth resuscitation. They are available in many community settings as well as in the hospital (and they are inexpensive so you may wish to buy one to keep in your car or carry with you). Some of them have ports to which you can connect an oxygen supply to increase the percentage of oxygen delivered by your breaths. They have an air-filled rim to allow a firm seal around the patient's nose and mouth. If you have to use one of these to resuscitate an infant, you can turn it upside down in order to get a better seal. *See Fig. 5.11.*

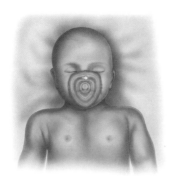

Figure 5.11 Using a pocket mask upside down for infants to get a better seal.

■ **Bag-valve-mask ventilation**. This equipment is available in each resuscitation bay in most hospitals and on the CRASH TROLLEY.

– **When to use it**. This can be used instead of a mouth-to-mouth technique when delivering Basic Life Support ventilations if there are other people helping you. If you are on your own then it will take too long to switch between compressions and ventilations if you try to use this method and you should instead stick to using mouth-to-mouth techniques until help arrives. If you are ventilating a child who does not need chest compressions then ventilate at a rate of 12–20 breaths per minute.

– **Attach an appropriately sized mask** to the bag and connect it to the oxygen supply. For children, a triangular-shaped mask can be used whereas for babies a circular mask often allows you to form a better seal and a T-piece is often used instead of a bag-valve-mask to allow ease of ventilation (see *Chapter 9 – Neonates for more detail*).

– **Form a tight seal** with the mask around the child's nose and mouth and keep the airway open as you give ventilations. Make sure that the cuff around the edge of the mask is inflated with air (use a syringe to do this if it is not already inflated) and press down only on the firm part of the mask (not the air-filled cuff) in order to gain a good seal against the child's face.

– **Use the c-shape technique if alone**. If you are the only person available to manage airway and breathing, you can deliver ventilation on your own. Use one hand to hold the mask onto the child's face and the other to squeeze the bag to deliver ventilation. This can require some practice to get right. With the hand holding the mask, form a c-shape with your thumb and forefinger and press down with the sides of these fingers onto the firm part of the mask. Then place your ring finger and little finger under the angle of the jaw and pull forwards towards the mask. This allows you to form a tight seal and helps to keep the airway open by lifting the lower jaw. Make sure that you have the appropriate amount of head tilt (as long as there is no suspicion of cervical spine injury) to keep the airway open. See *Fig. 5.12*.

– **Two-person technique is more effective**. If there are enough people present then the two-person technique can be much more effective, particularly

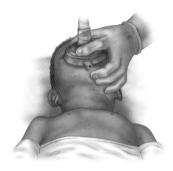

Figure 5.12 C-shape technique for hold on a bag-valve-mask for ventilation.

if you are inexperienced. To do this, one of you uses two hands to hold the mask in place whilst the other squeezes the bag to deliver ventilation. The person holding the mask can either use the c-shape technique but with both hands or use the heels of both thumbs to press down on the mask whilst using the fingers under the angles of the jaw on both sides to do a jaw thrust manoeuvre. *See Fig. 9.4 in Chapter 9 – Neonates.*

– **Watch to make sure that the chest rises and falls** as you deliver each ventilation. If it does not then read-just the head tilt (as long as there is no cervical spine injury) and make sure you have a tight seal with the mask before try-ing again.

Circulation management

In a child who has had a respiratory or cardiac arrest, the most important thing is to start effective Basic Life Support, so if you are in doubt about further man-

agement, continue with this until further help arrives. If you are confident and have been trained how to use a defibril-lator and resuscitation drugs then you may wish to start Advanced Life Support for management of a cardiac arrest.

■ **Put on the electrode pads**. Dry the child first if they are wet. Position one electrode over the apex of the heart (just below the nipple in the midclavicular line) and one just below the right clavicle or in an infant, place one pad on the back below the left scapula and one on the chest, to the left of the sternum. *See Fig. 5.13.*

■ **Automated devices**. If you are using an automated device it will instruct you as to whether or not to deliver a shock.

■ **Manual devices**. To use a manual device, you need to be able to interpret whether the child is in a shockable or non-shockable rhythm.

■ **Drugs**. Which drugs are given and when will depend on whether the child's heart is in a shockable or non-shockable rhythm.

Training in advanced resuscitation using defibrillators and medications in chil-dren who have had a cardiac arrest is provided on paediatric Advanced Life Support courses. A brief summary is available to download for free from the Resuscitation Council website (www. resus.org.uk). *See also Fig. 5.10 for a pae-diatric Advanced Life Support algorithm.*

Emergency drugs

Whereas in adult Advanced Life Support there is one set dose for each of the emergency drugs used, with children this

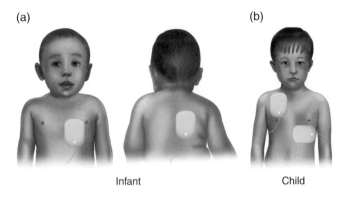

(a)   (b)

Infant   Child

Figure 5.13 Defibrillator pad positioning for infant (a) and child (b).

is obviously not possible because you would not give the same dose to a 9 month old as to a 12 year old. Doses are calculated by weight but in an emergency situation you may not have a recent weight for the child available so instead there are formulas that can be used to estimate a child's weight based on their age (see Table 5.1). Obviously if you have a recent actual weight for the child this is more accurate and you should use this instead.

 Top Tip

Remember never to exceed the adult dose when prescribing drugs by weight (see Table 5.1 for maximum doses of emergency drugs). This normally means giving adult doses to children who weigh over 40 kg.

You would never be expected to perform advanced management of a car-

diac arrest by yourself or lead a resuscitation as a junior member of the team. However, it can be useful to know the formulas used in a paediatric resuscitation so that you can start doing some of the calculations for common drugs that may need to be used. Many resuscitation rooms will have a whiteboard or something similar so that you can write the formulas up for everyone else to see. *Go to www. wileyhandsonguides.com/paediatrics for a small printable version of these formulas that you can attach to your ID badge.*

 Top Tip

There are often lots of people at a paediatric resuscitation. If there are already plenty of well-qualified people there helping, one of the most useful things you can do is to keep time and to document everything that happens. This is very rarely done well at resuscitations but an accurate record of exactly what has been done is crucial for providing a thorough handover to the transport team if the child needs to go to a TERTIARY CENTRE for intensive care (or even in handing over care to the intensive care team at your own hospital). It can be enormously helpful to the person leading the resuscitation to be able to check with you exactly how many doses of which drugs have been given and when. Also, record in the notes who is there, what their job title is and what time they arrive at the resuscitation so that it is possible to contact the relevant individuals later if necessary.

A commonly used mnemonic for calculations needed for a paediatric resuscitation is WET FLAG. See Table 5.1 for details. It is also possible to download a chart with precalculated doses of emergency medications for children of different ages from the Resuscitation Council website (www.resus.org.uk). You may wish to print out a copy to keep on your resuscitation trolley if one is not already available or to stick on the wall in resuscitation rooms.

ABCDE approach

See Fig. 5.14 for an algorithm of the structured approach to management of a sick child.

Regardless of the specific situation, it is really important to take a systematic approach to the management of an acutely unwell child. This allows you to make sure that you address any potential problems in the order of most urgent priority and avoids you missing anything. When using this approach, never move on to the next step until you have dealt with any problems identified in the earlier systems. This can be hard to stick to sometimes but is really important. For example, if a child has a wound that is bleeding it can be tempting to deal with this first but if they are unconscious and their airway is occluded, this will kill them much more quickly than the bleeding and must be dealt with first. The 'A–E' system for approaching resuscitation is well established and is taught on both paediatric and adult emergency life support courses. It is a simple way of remembering what you have to do. The letters stand for: Airway, Breathing, Circulation, Disability, Exposure.

A – Airway

The most urgent thing to assess in any emergency situation is whether air is able to travel effectively in and out of the trachea. Problems can occur in the oropharynx or the trachea itself.

Airway assessment
■ **Is the child able to talk or cry?**

■ **Are there any additional sounds?** Listen for any evidence of stridor or sturtor. These are squeaking or snoring noises as the child breathes in caused by a turbulent airflow as a result of partial airway occlusion. The volume of the noise is not an indication of the severity of obstruction.

Table 5.1 Calculations for commonly used emergency drugs

	Indication	Formula	Maximum dose
Weight (kg)	For calculation of drug doses	**Child 0–12 months** Weight = (0.5 × age in months) + 4 **Child 1–5 years** Weight = (2 × age in years) + 8 **Child 6–12 years** Weight = (3 × age in years) + 7	
Energy (J)	For delivery of asynchronous shock using a defibrillator	4 joules/kg	150–200 J biphasic for 1st shock 150–360 J biphasic for subsequent shocks
Tube size (internal diameter in mm, *uncuffed* tube)	For intubation	**Preterm babies** may need a 2.5 mm tube **Babies** usually require 3 or 3.5 mm tube **Children over 1 year**, tube size = (age in years/4) + 4	
Fluid bolus (IV or IO)	If showing signs of shock	10 mL/kg of 0.9% saline in trauma or DKA 20 mL/kg of 0.9% saline in all other circumstances	500 mL per bolus of 0.9% saline in trauma or DKA 1000 mL per bolus of 0.9% saline
Lorazepam (IV or IO)	To terminate seizures	100 micrograms/kg	Maximum single dose 4 mg
Adrenaline (IV or IO)	For cardiac arrest	10 micrograms/kg (0.1 mL/kg of 1:10,000 strength)	Maximum single dose 1 mg
Glucose 10% (IV or IO)	For hypoglycaemia	2–5 mL/kg of 10% dextrose	150–160 mL of 10% dextrose (over 10–15 mins)

Formulae from Advanced Life Support Group (2011) *Advanced Paediatric Life Support*. Wiley-Blackwell, Oxford.
DKA, diabetic ketoacidosis; IO, intraosseous; IV, intravenous.

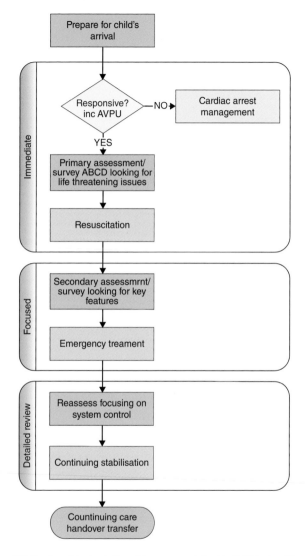

Figure 5.14 Algorithm of structured approach to management of a sick child. Reproduced from Advanced Life Support Group (2011) Advanced Paediatric Life Support, 5th edn. with permission of John Wiley & Sons, Ltd.

■ **Are they showing any signs of see-saw breathing?** This is when the chest is drawn in and the abdomen pushes out as the child attempts to breathe in against a closed airway.

■ **Is the child conscious?** If a child is unconscious then the tongue can fall back and occlude the airway and if they vomit then stomach contents can be inhaled.

■ **Look, listen and feel**. Place your cheek next to the child's mouth and see if you can feel their breath on your cheek, hear any breath sounds or see any movement of the chest. *If you can't see, hear or feel any evidence of breathing start Basic Life Support*.

Airway management (unconscious child)

■ *If a child is unconscious, commence the steps of Basic Life Support, making use of additional techniques mentioned in the Advanced Life Support section if equipment is available*.

Airway management (conscious child)

■ **Treat the underlying cause**. In cases of anaphylaxis the child will need to be given a dose of intramuscular (IM) adrenaline (*see full details on the management of anaphylaxis on page 113*). Nebulised adrenaline can be given in cases of croup in order to reduce some of the oedema of the mucosal layer lining the trachea.

 Top Tip

Be aware that with all observations, a value that falls within normal range definitely doesn't always mean that the child is well. The *trend* of the results is really important to look at and is much more meaningful than any isolated measurements. For example, a child may have had a heart rate that is within the normal range for the past 3 h but looking at the trend reveals that their heart rate has been gradually increasing over this time and is now at the upper limit of normal. This is really important to recognise as it indicates that the child may be developing signs of shock. Spotting this early allows you to intervene early. This is extremely important in children as they can compensate for illness for a long time and then deteriorate very rapidly. Looking at the entire clinical picture is also crucial when interpreting observations. For example, a child may have had a raised respiratory rate that has now normalised. This may either mean that the child has improved or be a very worrying sign that they are tiring and are no longer able to continue breathing quickly. Look at all the different observations together and examine the child for clinical signs before you make a judgement.

■ **Don't upset them**. If a child has partial occlusion of their airway but is still conscious, the last thing you want to do is make them start crying as this can make the airway obstruction even worse and cause them to decompensate. Avoid taking bloods or putting in a cannula and certainly don't try to examine the throat until you have senior colleagues present to help you (including an anaesthetist and an ENT surgeon in case the child totally occludes their airway and needs either intubation or a surgical airway).

■ **Give oxygen**. If the child can tolerate it, give 15 litres of oxygen through a non-rebreathe mask. This means that any air which is getting through to the lungs contains a much higher concentration of oxygen. In very small children who are upset by having a mask fitted, do not force them to wear a mask but instead ask their parents to hold it near their face (this is sometimes referred to as '**WAFTING OXYGEN**').

B – Breathing

Once you are happy that the child's airway is secure, you can move on to assessing breathing. In any child who is acutely unwell, put on an oxygen mask if they are able to tolerate it as a matter of course. This is because, regardless of the cause, if they are acutely unwell then they are likely to have an increased oxygen requirement and therefore giving a higher concentration of inhaled oxygen can help increase supply to the tissues.

Breathing assessment
■ **What is the child's respiratory rate?** Count the respiratory rate for 1 min and then refer to a table or observation chart to see if this is a normal rate for that child's age (see Table 5.2). *A table of normal observation values for children of different ages, which you can print and attach to your ID badge, is also available at www.wileyhandsonguides.com/paediatrics.* Don't be falsely reassured by a normal respiratory rate if the child is simultaneously tachycardic and looks very unwell; it may be that they are tiring and unable to breathe as quickly. This is a really worrying sign. If the child's respiratory rate is very low or they are not breathing at all, you will need to ventilate the lungs for them with bag-valve-mask ventilation.

■ **What are their oxygen saturation levels?** If a child has cold

Table 5.2 Normal observation values at different ages

	Age of child (years)				
	<1	1–2	2–5	5–12	>12
Respiratory rate	30–40	25–35	25–30	20–25	15–20
Heart rate	110–160	100–150	95–140	80–120	60–100
Systolic blood pressure	80–90	85–95	85–100	90–110	100–120

From Advanced Life Support Group (2011) *Advanced Paediatric Life Support.* Wiley-Blackwell, Oxford.

peripheries it can sometimes be difficult to get an accurate oxygen saturation reading from their finger. In some cases you may be able to get one from placing the probe on their big toe or ear lobe instead. If you record an oxygen saturation reading in the notes or on the observation chart, you must always record how much oxygen the child was breathing at the time otherwise the reading is meaningless. If a child has oxygen saturations of 93% in room air then you would be much less concerned than if this same reading was taken whilst they were breathing oxygen at 15 L/min, which would be very worrying. Treatment with oxygen should be started if oxygen saturation levels are below 92%. You should also give oxygen, even if the child's saturation levels are over 92%, if the child is tiring or they have increased work of breathing.

■ **Is the child showing any signs of respiratory distress?** Signs of respiratory distress include using any of the accessory muscles to assist the child in achieving adequate ventilation.

– **Head bobbing**. In small children and babies their head will bob up and down in time with their breathing if they are working very hard.

– **Subcostal recession**. This is when you can see an indrawing of the tissues under the lowest rib as the child breathes in.

– **Intercostal recession**. This is when you can see an indrawing of the soft tissue between the ribs as the child breathes in, making the ribs appear more prominent.

– **Sternal recession**. In young babies who are having great difficulty breathing, you may see the whole of the sternum being drawn inwards as the child breathes in.

– **Nasal flaring**. Flaring of the nostrils also indicates respiratory distress. This can be relatively subtle so look carefully.

– **Grunting**. This is exactly as the name describes, a small grunting noise as the child breathes out which is caused by them partially closing their airway in order to generate a positive pressure in the lungs to prevent airway collapse at the end of expiration. This is a sign of severe respiratory distress and is most often seen in babies.

– **Tracheal tug**. The trachea looks as if it is being tugged downwards as the child breathes in because they are using the strap muscles of their neck to assist them with breathing. Infants and toddlers have very short necks so you will need to get them to look up so that you can see the trachea.

■ **Is the chest wall moving symmetrically?** When you are observing the child's breathing to look for signs of respiratory distress, also look to check if the child's chest wall is moving symmetrically. If one side is moving much less than the other this may suggest a pneumothorax, pleural effusion or collapse on that side.

■ **Can you hear breath sounds?** Listen to the child's chest and ensure that you can hear good air entry throughout both lungs. Reduced breath sounds on one side could mean a pneumothorax or pleural effusion of that lung. Reduced breath sounds on both sides is an extremely worrying sign as this means that they are failing to get much air at all in and out of the lungs; this is called a 'silent chest' and is a sign of life-threatening asthma. *For more information on the management of acute asthma see page 115.*

■ **Can you hear additional sounds?** Is there any wheezing audible? Can you hear bronchial breathing or crackles? If the child has a lot of secretions in the upper airways, these noises can be transmitted so that they sound as if they are coming from the lungs. If this is the case then the sounds should improve or disappear completely for a while after the child coughs and clears their throat.

■ **Is there a normal percussion note?** Percuss both sides of the chest to assess for any altered percussion note. Hyperresonance may suggest a pneumothorax and dullness may indicate a pleural effusion, consolidation or haemothorax.

■ **Does the child look pale or cyanotic?** Hypoxia causes pallor of the skin around the lips. If there is evidence of central cyanosis (i.e. a blueish-purple colour to the lips and surrounding skin) then this is a preterminal sign and suggests that the child is imminently about to have a respiratory arrest.

Breathing management
■ **Give high-flow oxygen**. Give oxygen via a facemask at a sufficient concentration to maintain the oxygen saturations above 92%.

■ **Support breathing if low respiratory rate**. If a child's respiratory rate is low, they will need to be ventilated using a bag-valve-mask. Start the Basic Life Support protocol and use additional techniques mentioned in the Advanced Life Support section if you have access to appropriate equipment. ***Put out a crash call (2222) or call the emergency services (999) for any child who is requiring ventilation***.

■ **Treat urgent respiratory problems**.

– **Tension pneumothorax**. This requires immediate decompression. Signs suggestive of a tension pneumothorax include reduced chest movement unilaterally, reduced breath sounds unilaterally, hyperresonance unilaterally, distended neck veins, shock and trachea deviated away from the side of pneumothorax (late sign). To decompress, insert a wide-bore cannula in the midclavicular line in the second intercostal space. Aim just above the top edge of the lower rib in order to avoid the neurovascular bundle that runs along the bottom edge of each rib. You should hear a hissing noise as air is released through the needle. Needle decompression is a temporary emergency measure to relieve a tension pneumothorax but the child will also need insertion of a chest drain to prevent air from accumulating again.

– **Wheeze**. A brief history is important here to help determine the underlying cause to allow more definitive management (e.g. is this asthma or bronchiolitis or an inhaled foreign body?). However, bronchodilators are likely to be helpful in most situations of wheeze. Try a *salbutamol nebuliser*

(2.5 mg for children under 5 years, 5 mg over 5 years) and consider also giving *ipratropium bromide nebuliser* (125 micrograms if under 5 years, 250 micrograms if over 5 years).

C – Circulation

Once you have secured the airway, put on oxygen and assessed breathing and dealt with any issues you have found, you can move on to assessing the circulation.

Circulation assessment

■ **Does this child have warm peripheries?** Cold hands and feet may be a sign that the child has shut down their peripheral circulation in order to maintain perfusion of their vital organs. If a child has a severely compromised circulation, you may notice that the skin feels cold not just on the feet but also over their lower legs. There are certain kinds of shock that can result in the child having warm peripheries despite having a reduced apparent circulating volume. For more about the different kinds of shock, see below.

■ **What is their capillary refill time?** This should be assessed using a central location to give a more accurate assessment of the circulation (as peripheral CAPILLARY REFILL TIME may be reduced as a normal reaction in a cold room). Press down firmly on the skin over the sternum for 5 sec then remove your finger and count how long it takes for that area of skin to go back to a normal colour (initially the skin should appear blanched when you first remove your finger). A normal central CAPILLARY REFILL TIME is anything less than 2 sec for the skin to

return to a normal colour. Any longer than this suggests a circulatory problem. Don't forget to document the number of seconds as well as the fact that it is prolonged in order for other people reading it to appreciate the degree of severity.

■ **What is their heart rate?** Tachycardia can be a sign of circulatory shock. Although a child's heart rate will be elevated slightly when they are crying, if their pulse is persistently elevated this may suggest a circulatory problem. *If a child's heart rate is less than 60 beats per minute or rapidly falling with associated fall in blood pressure then this is a preterminal sign and you should start Basic Life Support and put out a crash call (2222) or call emergency services (999)*.

■ **What do their pulses feel like?** If you are unable to feel a child's peripheral pulses or they have weak central pulses then this is a sign of severe shock. A child with sepsis, hypercapnia or some types of congenital structural heart defects may have 'bounding pulses' that can be felt very strongly peripherally and centrally.

■ **What is their blood pressure?** Children are very good at maintaining their blood pressure within normal range and can compensate for large volume losses. Do not be reassured by a child who has a normal blood pressure as this is one of the last things to change and if it drops, this is a sign that the child will rapidly deteriorate and cardiac arrest may be imminent. When measuring the child's blood pressure, it is vital to use the correct size of cuff in order to get an accurate reading. The cuff should be over 80% of the length of the child's upper arm and the bladder of the cuff over 40% of the child's arm upper arm circumference.

■ Is there fluid loss or fluid in the wrong place?

Fluid loss   Shock as a result of fluid loss is known as hypovolaemic shock. Children with hypovolaemic shock will show signs of 'cold shock' (see Table 5.3). Examples of diagnoses that can result in shock due to fluid loss include:

■ blood loss

■ vomiting and diarrhoea

■ burns.

Fluid in the wrong place   Peripheral dilation of blood vessels and increased seepage of fluid from the blood vessels into the tissues can result in shock. These children may have a normal volume of fluid in their bodies but it has either leaked into the soft tissues, meaning that there is insufficient volume left in the blood vessels, or their peripheral blood vessels are all dilated, meaning that they have to use

other mechanisms (such as tachycardia) to maintain their cardiac output. These children will show signs of 'warm shock' (see Table 5.3). Examples of diagnosis that can result in fluid in the wrong place are:

■ anaphylaxis

■ sepsis.

■ Is this compensated or uncompensated shock?

COMPENSATED SHOCK   This means that the child is managing to maintain perfusion to their vital organs despite having underlying shock due to use of their body's compensatory mechanisms. The body maintains cardiac output by increasing heart rate and the child will also have a raised respiratory rate in order to compensate for the metabolic acidosis that results from shock. Depending on the underlying cause, the child may exhibit different signs of either warm shock or cold shock. *See Table 5.3 for signs of warm and cold shock.* See Fluid

Table 5.3 Signs present in warm shock and cold shock

Warm shock	Cold shock
Agitation, drowsiness or unconsciousness	Agitation, drowsiness or unconsciousness
Tachycardia	Tachycardia
Tachypnoea	Tachypnoea
Decreased urine output	Decreased urine output
Clammy, warm extremities	Cool hands and feet
Flushed, red skin	Pale or mottled skin
Flash capillary refill	Prolonged CAPILLARY REFILL TIME
Bounding peripheral pulses	Weak peripheral pulses
Normal/high systolic blood pressure	Normal/high systolic blood pressure
Low diastolic blood pressure	Normal/high diastolic blood pressure
Wide pulse pressure	Narrow pulse pressure

loss versus Fluid in the wrong place above for underlying diagnoses.

DECOMPENSATED SHOCK *If a child is showing signs of decompensated shock, put out a paediatric arrest call to get help rapidly.* A child who has previously been managing to compensate for shock may tire and decompensate. Decompensated shock can rapidly deteriorate into a respiratory or cardiac arrest without proper intervention so make sure that you get senior input immediately. Signs of decompensated shock include:

■ hypotension

■ decreased level of consciousness

■ anuria

■ bradycardia (preterminal sign, start Basic Life Support).

Circulation management

■ **Gain access.** Try to gain intravenous access if possible but do not spend a long time on multiple attempts. If intravenous access is not proving immediately possible in an acutely unwell child, attempt intraosseous access instead. *See Chapter 6 – Practical Procedures, for details.*

■ **Take blood samples.** As you gain intravenous or intraosseous access, draw back on the cannula or intraosseous needle to obtain a blood sample. If you have taken a sample from an intraosseous needle, this is bone marrow rather than blood and can only be used for restricted tests and never in a blood gas machine. *See Chapter 6 – Practical Procedures, for more details or call your hospital laboratory for advice.*

■ **If shocked, give a bolus of 0.9% saline.** The volume of fluid to give will depend on the underlying cause. In most cases of shock a bolus of 20 mL/kg of 0.9% saline is appropriate, repeated as necessary until clinical signs improve. If you suspect an underlying diagnosis of diabetic ketoacidosis, hyponatraemia or heart failure you should give a bolus of 10 mL/kg of 0.9% saline.

Top Tip

If you are treating a young baby who is not responding to your treatment for shock or who is cyanosed despite oxygen therapy, consider an underlying diagnosis of duct-dependent congenital heart disease. If this is the case, giving a prostaglandin can keep the duct patent and prevent any further deterioration. This should not be done without senior supervision. There is a detailed guideline on duct-dependent congenital cardiac disease on the CATS website for reference (www.cats.nhs.uk).

D – Disability

Once you have managed airway, breathing and circulation and are happy that these are stable for now, you can move on to assess disability. This means assessing neurological function and has several different components.

Disability assessment

■ **What is this child's conscious level?** The Glasgow Coma Scale is often used in adults but less frequently used in children, apart from in severe head injury (see *Table 5.4 for age-specific Glasgow Coma Scale*). In most paediatric emergency situations, the AVPU assessment tends to be used instead as part of the initial assessment. AVPU stands for:

– **A**lert
– responds to **V**oice
– responds only to **P**ain
– **U**nresponsive.

Any child who has a conscious level of P or U will be unable to protect their own airway and intubation should be considered. To assess response to pain,

either squeeze the child's trapezius muscle firmly or apply pressure to the bony supraorbital area, just below the inner aspect of the eyebrow (being careful not to press on the eyeball).

■ **Are their pupils of equal size and reactive?** Check to make sure that the pupils are the same size as each other and both respond to light. Pupils of markedly different sizes or that fail to constrict when you shine a light in them may indicate a serious underlying brain disorder.

■ **What is the child's posture?** DECORTICATE and DECEREBRATE postur-

Table 5.4 Glasgow Coma Scale for Children

Glasgow Coma Scale (>4 years)	Glasgow Coma Scale (<4 years)
Eye opening	***Eye opening***
4 Spontaneously	4 Spontaneously
3 To verbal stimuli	3 To verbal stimuli
2 To pain	2 To pain
1 No response to pain	1 No response to pain
Best motor response	***Best motor response***
6 Obeys verbal command	6 Spontaneous or obeys verbal command
5 Localises to pain	5 Localises to pain or withdraws to touch
4 Withdraws from pain	4 Withdraws from pain
3 Abnormal flexion to pain (decorticate)	3 Abnormal flexion to pain (decorticate)
2 Abnormal extension to pain (decerebrate)	2 Abnormal extension to pain (decerebrate)
1 No response to pain	1 No response to pain
Best verbal response	***Best verbal response***
5 Oriented and converses	5 Alert; babbles, coos words to ability
4 Disoriented and converses	4 Fewer than usual words, spontaneous irritable cry
3 Inappropriate words	3 Cries only to pain
2 Incomprehensible sounds	2 Moans to pain
1 No response to pain	1 No response to pain

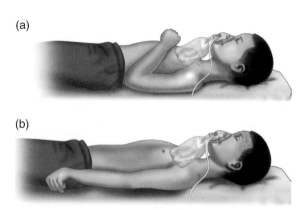

(a)

(b)

Figure 5.15 Decorticate (a) and decerebrate (b) posturing.

ing can both indicate severe underlying brain pathology. DECORTICATE POSTURING is when the child is stiff and has their arms flexed and their legs extended. DECEREBRATE POSTURING is when the child is stiff and has both their arms and legs extended. These postures can sometimes be mistaken for seizures. *See Fig. 5.15 for illustrations of decorticate and decerebrate posturing.*

■ **What is the child's blood glucose level?** Some people remember this by thinking about 'DEFG' after ABC to stand for Don't Ever Forget Glucose. It is particularly important to check a blood glucose level in a child who is fitting or with altered conscious level as it is an easily reversible cause.

Disability management
■ **Treat hypoglycaemia**. If the child is unconscious give 2–5 mL/kg of intravenous 10% dextrose. If intravenous access has not been possible, you can

given an intramuscular injection of glucagon (500 micrograms if <8 years or body weight <25kg, 1 mg if >8 years or 25 kg). If the child is conscious and able to swallow safely, you can give 100 mL fruit juice or 2–3 dextrose tablets followed by a complex carbohydrate such as a piece of toast or a bowl of cereal.

E – Exposure

Once you have assessed and managed airway, breathing, circulation and disability, you can move on to exposure. This means assessing two things.

■ **What is the child's temperature?** This needs to be assessed as a fever may indicate an underlying infection. Similarly, it is important to check for hypothermia and to keep the child warm during resuscitation.

■ **Do they have any rashes?** Look systematically at all the child's skin. Is there evidence of any rashes? For example, petechiae may indicate septicaemia, bruises may suggest child abuse or urticaria may be present in allergic reactions.

Reassess

At all stages during management of an acutely unwell child you must remember to keep reassessing the situation. Start from the beginning each time and reassess systematically A through to E.

Take a brief history

Once you have performed your initial assessment and resuscitation, you will need to take a focused history and perform a more thorough examination of the child as part of your secondary assessment. You do not have time to take a full history in the normal way but need to find out key pieces of information in order to inform your ongoing urgent management. There are some specific questions listed under the individual diagnosis sections below but the mnemonic AMPLE is a reminder for questions to ask in all cases.

■ **Allergies**. Does the child have any known allergies? Common triggers include food (especially nuts and shellfish), medication (especially penicillin, anaesthetic agents and contrast media for imaging), latex and insect stings.

■ **Medications**. Does the child take any regular medications? What are the names, doses and frequency? Have they been taking these medications as prescribed?

■ **Past medical history**. Any significant illnesses or accidents in the past requiring admissions to hospital? Any previous operations? Any long-term conditions?

■ **Last meal**. When did the child last have anything to eat or drink? This allows you to assess the risk of aspiration if the child needs anaesthesia and intubation (this is therefore particularly important in trauma cases).

■ **Events**. What happened leading up to the illness or injury? Any signs or symptoms over the preceding days or hours?

Anaphylaxis

Anaphylaxis is a potentially life-threatening allergic reaction, although death from this in children is very rare (one child a year in the UK). Symptoms can develop very rapidly (over minutes) and prompt treatment is needed. Individuals who have a history of severe allergic reaction will often carry an automatic device prefilled with adrenaline (such as EpiPen, Jext or Anapen) so that they can be given intramuscular adrenaline in the community as soon as their symptoms start.

History

Ask about:

■ ingestion of food containing known allergen (may be unknown if first presentation)

■ insect bite or sting (particularly bees and wasps)

■ new medications ingested or used topically for first time

- anaesthetic drug or contrast medium given

- rapid onset of symptoms

- previous severe allergic reaction

- history of asthma.

Symptoms

- Preceding itching and facial swelling
- Difficulty breathing
- Abdominal pain
- Diarrhoea

Signs

- Stridor
- Wheeze
- Face and tongue swelling
- Urticaria
- Hypotension
- Tachycardia

Immediate management

Remove allergen if still present.

- **Airway**

– *If the child has stridor or difficulty breathing, put out a paediatric crash call as they may need intubation or a surgical airway if they develop complete airway obstruction.*

– Give **intramuscular adrenaline 1:1000 (1 mg/mL)** at the correct dose for age (see Table 5.5) into the anterolateral aspect of the thigh.

– If child remains hypotensive, tachycardic, has stridor or difficulty breathing, a repeat dose of intramuscular adrenaline should be given after 5 min.

– **Consider nebulised adrenaline driven by oxygen** at 400 micrograms/kg (0.4 mL/kg of 1:1000) if the child still has stridor after the first dose of intramuscular adrenaline has been given. Max dose 5mg (5ml 1:1000)

- **Breathing**

– Give **high-flow oxygen** via non-rebreathe mask.

– **If child not breathing, start Basic Life Support**.

– If very wheezy, consider giving **nebulised salbutamol** (2.5 mg for under 5 years, 5 mg over 5 years).

- **Circulation**

– If shocked, give **20 mL/kg bolus of 0.9% saline**.

– **Lie patient flat and raise their legs**.

Table 5.5 Intramuscular adrenaline doses for use in anaphylaxis

Age	Volume of 1 in 1000 (1 mg/mL) adrenaline	Dose
<6 years	0.15 mL	150 micrograms
6–12 years	0.3 mL	300 micrograms
12–18 years	0.5 mL	500 micrograms

Table 5.6 Doses for chlorphenamine and hydrocortisone in anaphylaxis

Age	Chlorphenamine (IM or slow IV)	Hydrocortisone (IM or slow IV)
>12 years	10 mg	200mg
6–12 years	5 mg	100 mg
<6 years	2.5 mg	50 mg
<6 months	250 micrograms/kg	25 mg

IM, intramuscular; IV, intravenous.

– **Give hydrocortisone by intramuscular or slow intravenous injection**; can also be used in preventing secondary reactions and starts to have an onset within 3–4 h of dose (see Table 5.6 for doses).

Continually reassess and call for help if no improvement or child deteriorating.

Further management

■ **Chlorphenamine by intramuscular or slow intravenous injection** can also be of use but has a slower onset of action than adrenaline (see Table 5.6 for doses).

■ **Admit for observation**. It is possible for children to have a secondary onset of anaphylaxis without further exposure to the allergen so they should be admitted for a period of observation.

■ **Take a complete history**. Once the acute situation has resolved, make sure that someone returns to the family to take a complete history. It is important to try to identify the allergen through discussion with the family so that they are able to avoid future exposure.

Long-term management

■ **Refer to an allergy specialist**. The child will need to be referred to an allergy specialist for possible allergy testing.

■ **Discharge with further oral medication**. You may wish to prescribe further oral doses of antihistamine and steroids for the next 3 days in order to reduce the possibility of a repeat reaction.

■ **Consider prescribing an EpiPen (or equivalent)**. If the child has had a severe anaphylactic reaction then they will need an automated device for injection of adrenaline in the community should they have a repeat reaction. The child and their family will need to be trained in how and when to use the device. *For a demonstration of how to use an EpiPen, see Video 2.*

Acute asthma

Asthma is a chronic inflammatory disease of the airways. Children with asthma can have acute exacerbations, which at their most severe can be life-threatening.

History

Ask about:

- preceding coryzal symptoms
- inhaler use
- oral steroids
- previous admissions to hospital with exacerbations
- previous intubation
- previous intensive care admissions.

Symptoms

- Cough
- Wheeze
- Breathlessness
- Chest tightness

Signs

Proper assessment of symptoms and signs is important as it allows you to classify the severity of the child's asthma as defined by the British Thoracic Society (see Table 5.7).

If the child has signs or symptoms from more than one category, always treat them as if it were the most severe (even if they have only one sign from that category).

 Top Tip

Although peak flow measurement features in the assessment of severe and life-threatening asthma, it is unlikely that children under 6 years of age or those who are very breathless will be capable of completing a reliable reading from peak flow measurement.

Immediate management

If a child has any features of life-threatening asthma, put out a paediatric arrest call.

- **Airway**

– Is the child's airway patent? If not, try airway manoeuvres or airway adjuncts and put out an arrest call if you haven't already.

- **Breathing**

– **Give oxygen** at a sufficient flow rate to maintain oxygen saturations between 94% and 98%.

– **Give inhaled bronchodilators**. These should be given 'back to back' (immediately one after the other), alternating between salbutamol and ipratropium until there is an improvement of the child's symptoms. This is sometimes referred to as BURST THERAPY. These should be given as oxygen-driven nebulisers. If you are in the community and there are no facilities available to give an oxygen-driven nebuliser, then give 10 puffs of salbutamol using a spacer with an inhaler. *See Table 5.8 for doses. See Chapter 6 – Practical Procedures for details of how to set up a nebuliser and use a spacer and inhaler.*

– **Give steroid therapy**. This can be given either orally or intravenously. It is better to use intravenous steroids for children who are very breathless and requiring continuous oxygen or who are vomiting. Steroids take 3–4 h to work so should be given early (within the first hour of presentation) to allow for benefit as soon as possible. *See Table 5.9 for doses.*

Table 5.7 Severe and life-threatening asthma symptoms and signs

Severe	Life-threatening
Oxygen saturations <92% in air Too breathless to talk or eat PEF 33–50% Use of accessory neck muscles	Oxygen saturations <92% in air plus any of: Silent chest Poor respiratory effort Altered consciousness Cyanosis Agitation PEF <33% of best or predicted

Age 2–5 years	Age >5 years	
■ Heart rate >140/min ■ Respiratory rate >40/min	■ Heart rate >125/min ■ Respiratory rate >30/min	

PEF, peak expiratory flow.

Table 5.8 Doses for nebulised salbutamol and ipratropium in acute asthma

Age	Salbutamol	Ipratropium bromide
Under 5 years	2.5 mg	250 micrograms
5–12 years	5 mg	250 micrograms
Over 12 years	5 mg	500 micrograms

Table 5.9 Steroid doses in acute severe asthma

Age	Oral prednisolone	Intravenous hydrocortisone
Under 2 years	1–2 mg/kg	4 mg/kg (or 25 mg if weight unknown)
2–5 years	20 mg	4 mg/kg (or 50 mg if weight unknown)
5–12 years	40 mg	4 mg/kg (or 100 mg if weight unknown)
Over 12 years	40–50 mg	4 mg/kg (or 100 mg if weight unknown)

■ Circulation

– **Gain intravenous access** and take off blood for full blood count, c-reactive protein, urea and electrolytes and BLOOD GAS analysis.

– **Intravenous infusions**. Additional intravenous medications such as salbutamol, aminophylline or magnesium sulphate can be given to children who are not responding to initial treatment but this should not be started without senior input.

– **Repeated blood gas measurement** can be useful for children who are responding poorly to initial treatment to help judge the need for intubation. A normal carbon dioxide level on the blood gas of a child with severe asthma is worrying – it should be low as a result of the child's raised respiratory rate and a normal result suggests inadequate ventilation and that the child may be tiring.

Further management

■ **Consider transfer to a specialist unit**. If the child is responding poorly to treatment they may need intubation and transfer to a paediatric intensive care unit. Have a discussion early with the relevant unit or transfer team in order to gain their advice and to find a bed. See *Critical Care Transfer Services section later in this chapter for details of regional paediatric intensive care transfer teams.*

■ **Regular inhaled bronchodilators**. Whilst in hospital, the child will need ongoing treatment with inhaled bronchodilators. The interval between these can be gradually increased depending on the child's response. This is sometimes referred to as 'STRETCHING'. Assess the child just before their next dose of inhaled bronchodilator is due and if they are free of symptoms and signs of respiratory distress, consider delaying their subsequent dose for an hour and reassess. As the child's oxygen requirement reduces, oxygen-driven nebulisers can be replaced with inhalers and a spacer for delivery of the medication. *See Chapter 6 – Practical Procedures for details of how to set up a nebuliser and use an inhaler and spacer.*

■ **Regular steroid treatment**. The child will need regular steroid treatment whilst in hospital. This is given every 6 h if intravenous hydrocortisone or as a single oral dose of prednisolone. Once the child is well enough to swallow medication, they should be switched from intravenous to oral steroids.

Long-term management

Before discharge you should:

■ **Check inhaler technique**. Poor knowledge about how to use inhalers properly may have contributed to the exacerbation and requirement to be admitted to hospital. Ensuring that children and their parents know how to use their inhalers properly is very important. *See Chapter 6 – Practical Procedures, for details on inhaler technique*

■ **Consider the need for preventer medications**. If the child is not already on an inhaled steroid, this could be started. In children over 5 years of age, addition of a regular inhaled long-acting beta-agonist such as salmeterol could be considered or in children under 5, consider adding a leukotriene receptor antagonist (such as montelukast). For the latest guidance on the stepwise management of chronic asthma, see the British Thoracic Society guidance at www.brit-thoracic.org.uk

■ **Arrange referral to a paediatric respiratory specialist**. If the child has had life-threatening features, failed to respond well to initial treatment or is having persistent attacks despite preventive treatment

■ **Arrange follow-up** with the patient's GP in the next couple of days and also in the paediatric asthma clinic within the following 1–2 months

■ A written asthma management plan. It is vital for children to have a clear written asthma management plan to take away with them on discharge from hospital. This needs to have clear instructions about symptoms and signs to look out for and what to do if any of these are present (in terms of doses of inhalers and how urgently and where to seek medical attention). This is extremely important so that children are seen by healthcare staff and interventions made before the exacerbation develops into a severe one.

Drowning

Drowning can be very distressing for parents and healthcare professionals alike. It is the third most common cause of accidental death in paediatric patients in the UK.

Starting early and effective Basic Life Support is key to survival. 70% of children survive drowning when Basic Life Support is given at the scene whereas only 40% survive without early Basic Life Support (Advanced Life Support Group 2011).

If the child is unconscious, put out a paediatric trauma call (2222) or call the emergency services (999) and start Basic Life Support if the child is showing no signs of life.

History

Ask about:

■ events leading to submersion

■ where and what kind of water: contaminated water/swimming pool/ temperature

■ duration of submersion

■ if any Basic Life Support was given at the scene

■ if the child quickly recovered consciousness.

Signs

■ Hypoxia

■ Hypothermia

■ Cardiac arrhythmia

■ Unconscious

Immediate management

■ Airway

– Open airway. You may need to use an airway adjunct to help keep the airway open initially whilst awaiting assistance from someone who is able to intubate. The child will need intubation to protect the airway as there is often a lot of water in the stomach which can result in aspiration without a definitive airway.

– Stabilise the cervical spine if you suspect injury. Use your hands to do this until you can find a collar to put on. If the child needs Basic Life Support, avoid using a head tilt and opt for a jaw thrust as first choice of airway manoeuvre instead.

■ Breathing

– Basic Life Support if needed. Look, listen and feel for 10 sec; if the child is not breathing then start Basic Life Support.

– Give oxygen. If the child is breathing spontaneously, give oxygen at sufficient concentration to keep the saturations at 94–98%.

■ Circulation

– **Defibrillation needed?** If a child is requiring Basic Life Support and someone arrives with an automated external defibrillator, make sure that you dry the skin before applying the electrode pads. Automated external defibrillators can assess the cardiac rhythm for you and will tell you whether or not to deliver a shock.

■ Disability

– **Assess conscious level and pupils** on admission as this can be useful for monitoring future progress or deterioration.

■ Exposure

– **Measure core temperature.** Children who have been submerged in water frequently develop hypothermia. Measure the child's core temperature using a rectal or oesophageal thermometer capable of recording low readings. Hypothermia (core body temperature of <35°C) can mimic death and cause cardiac arrhythmias. Although initial hypothermia may help with an element of neuroprotection, it can also cause cardiac arrhythmias refractory to defibrillation and the need for prolonged resuscitation.

– **Rewarm slowly**. Children who are hypothermic need to be rewarmed slowly (at a rate of 0.25–0.5°C per hour), meaning that resuscitation may have to continue for a prolonged period of time as defibrillation is unlikely to be effective if the child's core temperature

is less than 30°C and resuscitation efforts should not be stopped until the child's core temperature is at least 32°C.

– **Simple rewarming measures**. You will be easily able to do these yourself (but do not interrupt Basic Life Support to do this if you are on your own). Remove any wet clothes and cover the child with blankets. These measures are insufficient on their own for children in cardiac arrest and more sophisticated methods such as intravenous fluid warmed to 39°C, using warmed humidified oxygen and extracorporeal blood rewarming will need to be used by senior colleagues depending on what facilities are available.

Further management

■ Insert a nasogastric tube. Once
the child has been intubated, a nasogastric tube should be inserted to allow drainage of water from the stomach as it is usually full of water the child has swallowed.

■ Admit for observation. Children
can have a delayed deterioration in respiratory function following a drowning incident so, even if the child appears well, they should be admitted for observation for at least 8 h.

■ Monitor for signs of pneumonia.
There is no evidence that prophylactic antibiotics are helpful but the child must be monitored carefully for signs of aspiration pneumonia and broad-spectrum intravenous antibiotic treatment started if necessary.

■ Monitor for raised intracranial
pressure. Raised intracranial pressure

may develop after hypoxic brain injury as a result of drowning. Monitor for signs such as abnormal posture, tachycardia, dilated pupil(s) or papilloedema. **Bradycardia, hypertension and irregular respiration are late, pre-terminal signs**.

■ **Maintain normoglycaemia**. Blood glucose levels should be carefully monitored and well controlled in order to improve neurological outcome.

■ **Look for an underlying cause**. In some cases, the reason for drowning is obvious from the history but in an older child who is able to swim, look for potential underlying causes such as seizures or cardiac arrhythmias that resulted in the child losing consciousness whilst in the water.

Sepsis

Sepsis is very important to recognise but it can be difficult at times to differentiate between common childhood infections and the early stages of serious infections that require treatment with antibiotics. It is crucial to assess thoroughly any child presenting with fever for key signs and symptoms that may suggest developing sepsis in order to treat promptly and prevent deterioration. This is particularly important for children presenting with signs of shock as their risk of mortality will double for every hour that their septic shock remains untreated. Babies are at higher risk of serious infection and can present in a non-specific way.

History

Ask about:

■ fever

■ cough

■ rashes

■ headache

■ contact with others who are unwell

■ vomiting and diarrhoea

■ decreased urine output.

Symptoms and signs

Thorough assessment of symptoms and signs of sepsis is important to avoid missing any cases of potentially serious infection or to avoid overusing antibiotics in children who do not need them. The NICE guidelines on assessment of fever in children under the age of 5 categorises children into low, intermediate or high risk of serious infection based on the presence or absence of certain symptoms and signs (see NICE Clinical Guideline No. 47, available at www.nice.org.uk). Particularly concerning signs that suggest severe infection include the following.

■ A high fever in a young baby

– Temperature ≥38°C aged 0–3 months

– Temperature ≥39°C aged 3–6 months

■ Signs of respiratory distress

■ Reduced conscious level

■ Pale or mottled skin

■ Evidence of dehydration

■ Signs suggestive of a concerning underlying diagnosis, e.g. non-blanching rash, bulging fontanelle or bile-stained vomiting

Immediate management

■ **Airway**

– **Is the child's airway obstructed?**

– **Are they sufficiently conscious to protect their own airway?** Deal with any issues concerning the airway before moving on.

■ **Breathing**

– **Give oxygen** at sufficient concentration to maintain oxygen saturation levels at or above 95%. Even if there is not a primary respiratory cause for the child's illness, they will have an increased oxygen requirement as a result of the metabolic acidosis that occurs in sepsis.

■ **Circulation**

– **Obtain access.** Try to get intravenous access, ideally two separate lines. If you are having difficulty gaining access, do not waste valuable time but instead try to gain intraosseous access.

– **Take bloods as you insert access.** Take bloods for blood culture, full blood count, electrolytes, c-reactive protein, coagulation screen, group and save and venous blood gas to gain a further picture of the degree of hypoxia and lactate accumulation and for an immediate estimate of electrolytes.

– **Give a fluid bolus**. For any child showing signs of shock give an immediate bolus of **20 mL/kg of 0.9% saline over 5 min**.

– **Reassess** heart rate, CAPILLARY REFILL TIME, mental state and peripheral pulses and give further fluid boluses if necessary. A child may need up to 60 mL/kg of IV fluid boluses.

– **Give high-dose broad-spectrum antibiotics** such as ceftriaxone. For children aged over 1 month, this can be given at a dose of 80 mg/kg up to a maximum dose of 4 g daily. For babies less than 1 month old, a dose of 20–50 mg/kg once daily can be given as a slow infusion over 60 min.

– **Consider human albumin solution for further boluses**. Ideally, children who are still shocked after 40 mL/kg of 0.9% saline should be given 20 mL/kg boluses of 4.5% human albumin solution thereafter. If this is not readily available in your department then further boluses of 0.9% saline can be given but monitor closely for signs of fluid overload (fine inspiratory crackles at lung bases, hepatomegaly, gallop rhythm on auscultation of the heart, raised jugular venous pulse). If a child is requiring this much fluid and is still shocked, they are likely to need intubation and inotropes. ***Contact your local critical care transfer team at this stage if there is no paediatric intensive care unit at your hospital or involve the paediatric intensive care team at your own hospital***.

■ **Disability**

– **Correct hypoglycaemia**. Give 2 mL/kg of 10% dextrose intravenously to correct any hypoglycaemia.

Further management

Once the child is stable, consider performing further investigations in order to establish the underlying cause of the sepsis.

■ **Chest x-ray**. To look for any evidence of consolidation on the chest x-ray that might suggest pneumonia as the underlying cause for the sepsis.

■ **Lumbar puncture**. In older children who have signs of meningism (photophobia or headache), consider performing a lumbar puncture as long as there are no signs of raised intracranial pressure. *For more details see Chapter 6 – Practical Procedures.* In young babies and in children for whom no obvious source of infection has been found, lumbar puncture is important for diagnosis (even if taken after antibiotics have been given).

Meningococcal septicaemia

This is systemic septicaemia as a result of infection with *Neisseria meningitidis*. It is potentially fatal and if suspected needs to be treated promptly. Any child with a purpuric rash and a fever should be treated for meningococcal septicaemia unless you are certain of an alternative diagnosis. Do not be reassured by the absence of a purpuric rash as this is sometimes absent initially and once it develops, can spread rapidly (indicating underlying disseminated intravascular coagulation as a result of septicaemia).

History

Ask about:

■ headache

■ photophobia

■ rashes

■ irritability.

Symptoms

■ Headache

■ Photophobia

■ Lethargy

■ Reduced consciousness

■ Irritability

 Top Tip

Do not confuse the different terminology; meningitis is a different diagnosis from meningococcal septicaemia. Meningitis is a localised infection that can result from infection with a number of different bacteria or viruses. Meningococcal septicaemia is a systemic infection with *N. meningitidis* (a type of meningococcal bacteria) that results in sepsis. ***Many children with meningococcal septicaemia will not also have meningitis (and therefore no signs of meningism)***.

Signs

Signs of meningococcal septicaemia include:

■ fever

■ non-blanching (purpuric) rash

■ tachycardia

■ hypotension (late sign)

■ low platelets, low white cell count (do not wait for blood results, make diagnosis clinically if at all suspicious).

Initial management

■ Airway

– **Assess airway and protect if child unconscious**. If the child is unconscious they will need intubation to protect their airway. You can use airway adjuncts whilst you are waiting for experienced help to arrive.

■ Breathing

– **Give oxygen** at sufficient concentration to maintain saturations above 95%.

■ Circulation

– **Gain access quickly**. Ideally this should be two intravenous lines but if you are having difficulty gaining intravenous access, do not delay and try the intraosseous route instead.

– **Take blood samples** for culture, meningococcal polymerase chain reaction (PCR), full blood count, clotting function, urea and electrolytes, c-reactive protein and a venous gas (these can be taken from the line as it is inserted).

– **Give fluid bolus** of 20 mL/kg of 0.9% saline. Reassess signs of shock after first bolus and repeat if necessary up to 60 mL/kg in total.

– **Give 50mg/kg of Cefotaxime** intravenously or intraosseously. Maximum dose is 12 g daily.

■ Disability

– **Check level of consciousness and pupils**. If the child has a fluctuating level of consciousness, decorticate or DECEREBRATE POSTURING or seizures then suspect raised intracranial pressure. If

this is the case, **do not perform a lumbar puncture** and consider giving an infusion of 3 mL/kg of 3% saline.

> **Top Tip**
>
> Don't forget to inform the Health Protection Agency of any cases of suspected meningococcal septicaemia as this is a notifiable disease.

Burns and scalds

Put out a paediatric trauma call for children with severe burns or any burns to the face or mouth.

Children with burns should be treated in a specialist burns centre. You should discuss with your nearest burns centre and arrange for urgent transfer.

Burns can occur from contact with fire, heat, chemicals or electricity, scalds from contact with hot liquid.

History

Ask about:

- ■ mechanism of injury
- ■ timing of injury
- ■ smoke exposure
- ■ any first aid measures taken
- ■ any other injuries.

Symptoms

- ■ Partial-thickness burns are painful.
- ■ Full-thickness burns are painless.

Signs

- Erythema (superficial burns)
- Blisters, pink and speckled skin (partial-thickness burns)
- White or black leathery and painless skin (full-thickness burns)

Immediate management

■ Airway

– **Smoke inhalation injury?** A child who has been in a fire may also have damage to their airway from smoke inhalation. Oedema causes rapid deterioration of the airway so if you suspect smoke inhalation is even a possibility, *put out a paediatric trauma call as the child is likely to need tracheal intubation*. The longer you leave it, the more difficult intubation becomes because of the worsening oedema so if in any doubt, call a senior colleague or anaesthetist at the earliest possible opportunity.

– **Scalds or burns to face and mouth**. A child's airway can also be compromised by scalds or severe burns to their face or mouth so look specifically for these injuries and call for help early if they are present.

■ Cervical spine

– If there is any possibility of cervical spine injury from the history, place the child in a collar and blocks until this has been excluded.

■ Breathing

– **Give high-flow oxygen** at sufficient concentration to maintain saturations above 95%.

– **Assess for circumferential burns** to the chest or abdomen that may restrict chest movement and cause breathing difficulties. It may be necessary for an experienced member of staff to perform an escharotomy (incision through the burnt skin) in order to allow for adequate chest expansion.

■ Circulation

– **Gain access**. Put in two intravenous cannulae, avoiding placing them in areas of burnt skin if possible. If you are having difficulty gaining intravenous access, do not delay and instead gain intraosseous access.

– **Give a 20 mL/kg bolus of 0.9% saline** if the child is showing signs of shock. Children rarely show signs of shock as a result of burns in the first few hours so if this is the case, look carefully for other causes (such as internal bleeding).

– **Perform an electrocardiogram (ECG)** if there was an electrical cause for the burns.

■ Disability

– **Assess conscious level**. This is important as a baseline for future changes in consciousness.

– **Give adequate analgesia**. Burns can be extremely painful and the child may need opiate analgesia for pain.

■ Exposure

– **Keep warm**. Children with burns can get cold very quickly because of heat loss through their damaged skin. Make sure that they are covered with plenty of blankets and heated blankets too if necessary.

– **Check entirety of the skin** in order to calculate the percentage of body surface area involved.

– **Cover burns with clingfilm**. This can be used as a temporary dressing whilst awaiting transfer of the child to a specialist burns unit. Do not wrap the dressing all the way around a limb or the torso but instead place individual sheets loosely over burnt areas. Minimise disruptions once dressings have been applied and avoid unnecessary re-examination.

 Top Tip

There are different charts available for children of different ages to use when estimating percentage body surface area affected by burns. If you do not have charts available, you can estimate by comparing the area affected to the size of the child's hand (palm and fingers) which is equivalent to 1% of their body surface area. When estimating percentage body surface area affected by burns, include only areas of deep partial-thickness burns (which appear pale pink, speckled and blistered) or full-thickness burns (which appear pale in colour, or leathery and sometimes black). Do not include superficial burns (areas of erythematous skin that obviously blanch and rapidly refill).

Further management

■ **Prescribe additional intravenous fluids for children with burns covering more than 10% of their body surface area**. Children with burns to large areas of their skin will have additional fluid requirements due to the increased water loss from the damaged skin. Their additional fluid requirement should be added to their normal maintenance volume (see *Chapter 7 – Prescribing in Children, for details of how to calculate the normal maintenance fluid volume*). Their additional fluid requirements can be calculated using the following formula.

Additional fluid requirement
= % body surface area burnt
× weight (kg) × 4

Fluid requirement in child with
burns = maintenance + (% body
surface area × weight (kg) × 4)

■ Half of this fluid volume should be given over the first 8 h from the time of injury. The remaining half should be given over the following 16 h. This means that you will need to calculate different infusion rates for each prescription. You will also need to adjust the rate of infusion based on the child's clinical signs. See Box 5.1 for a worked example.

■ **Careful fluid balance monitoring**. In children with large areas of burns, fluid balance should be monitored closely and the child may need to be catheterised to allow for accurate assessment. Aim for a urine output of ≥1 mL/kg/h and adjust fluid infusion rates accordingly to achieve this.

Ongoing management

In the case of burns and scalds, you must always consider the possibility of these being deliberately inflicted

Box 5.1 Example of fluid prescription for a child with burns

A child is brought to the emergency department having been in a house fire. You have put out a paediatric trauma call and your seniors have intubated the child and completed initial stabilisation. He has not required any fluid boluses and has a normal heart rate and blood pressure. Your consultant asks you to prescribe intravenous fluids for the child.

You estimate that his burns cover 15% of his body surface area. The child is 6 years old but you do not have a recent weight for him.

■ **Estimate weight**

$$\text{Weight} = \text{age (in years)} + 4 \times 2 = (6 + 4) \times 2 = 20 \text{ kg}$$

■ **Calculate additional fluid requirements**

$$\text{Additional fluid requirement in ml} = \% \text{ body surface area burnt} \times \text{weight (kg)} \times 4 = 15 \times 20 \times 4 = 1200 \text{ mL}$$

■ **Calculate maintenance fluid** (*for details on how to do this, see Chapter 7 – Prescribing in Children*)

$$\text{Maintenance fluid} = (100 \times 10) + (50 \times 10) = 1500 \text{ mL}$$

■ **Calculate the rate of infusion.** Half of the *additional* fluid volume needs to be given over the first 8 h and half over the next 16 h.

Half of the additional fluid volume = 1200/2 = 600 mL to be given over 8 h. Therefore the rate of infusion would be 600/8 = 75 mL/h

Maintenance fluid to be given over 24 h, therefore the hourly rate is 1500/24 = 62.5 mL/h (round up to 63 mL/h)

So for the first 8 h the infusion rate of fluid should be 75 + 63 = 138 mL/h.

The next half of the additional fluid volume should be given over the subsequent 16 h so the rate of infusion at this stage will be 600/16 = 37.5 mL/h (round up to 38 mL/h).

So for the subsequent 16 h the infusion rate of fluid should be 38 + 63 = 101 mL/h.

rather than accidental. Take a thorough history of what happened and when, who was there and what was done immediately after the burn or scald happened. There are certain patterns of injury that are more likely to have been inflicted rather than accidental. *See Chapter 4 – Child Protection and Safeguarding, for more details.* Even if you think that the injury is accidental rather than inflicted, it is important to ensure that parents understand how to prevent future similar accidents from occurring and it may be sensible to arrange for the health visitor to see them at home following discharge. *If you have any concerns about the child's welfare, whether about inflicted injury or poor supervision allowing the accident to take place, it is crucial that you raise this with senior colleagues.*

Seizures

See Fig. 5.16 for an algorithm of the management of status epilepticus.

There are many different underlying causes for seizures that must be considered after initial resuscitation. The majority of seizures in childhood will resolve spontaneously after 5 min. If this is not the case then medication can be given at this stage.

Status epilepticus is defined as a generalised seizure lasting for longer than 30 min or multiple seizures over a period of 30 min without regaining consciousness between seizures.

History

Ask about:

- history of fever
- previous seizures
- known epilepsy
- compliance with antiepileptic medications
- head injury
- diabetes/inborn errors of metabolism
- preceding headache, photophobia or irritability
- hypoxic episode (drowning or preceding vasovagal episode)
- accidental or self-poisoning.

Immediate management

- **Airway**
  - **Try a nasopharyngeal airway**. If a child is having a prolonged generalised seizure, they are likely to have their jaw tightly clenched shut. If this is the case and you suspect airway compromise, you can use a nasopharyngeal airway adjunct to help open the airway.
- **Breathing**
  - **Give oxygen** at a rate of 15 L/min via a non-rebreathe mask.
- **Circulation**
  - **Gain intravenous access if possible**, in case medications need to be given to terminate the seizures.
- **Disability**
  - **Check blood glucose** and correct any hypoglycaemia with 2–5 mL/kg of 10% dextrose intravenously or intramuscular glucagon injection if

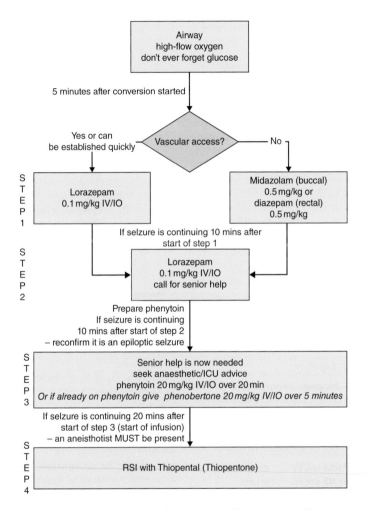

Figure 5.16 Algorithm for the management of status epilepticus. ICU, intensive care unit; IO, intraosseous; IV, intravenous; RSI, rapid sequence induction. Reproduced from Advanced Life Support Group (2011) Advanced Paediatric Life Support, 5th edn. with permission of John Wiley & Sons, Ltd..

intravenous access is not available. The dose of glucagon for intramuscular injection is 500 micrograms in children under 10 years or 1 mg in children over 10 years old.

– **Give a benzodiazepine** in an attempt to terminate the seizure if it continues for longer than 5 min or if the child appears to be in status epilepticus. Ideally this should be given intravenously but if no access is available you can use buccal or rectal routes for delivery. See Table 5.10 for doses and drugs of choice.

– **Repeat dose of benzodiazepine if needed**. If the child is still fitting 10 min after you have given the first dose of benzodiazepine, give a repeat dose.

– **Get senior help if still fitting after 20 min**. If the child continues to fit after two doses of benzodiazepines, you should get senior help if you haven't already as the child may need a phenytoin infusion or anaesthesia and intubation.

■ **Exposure**

– **Measure temperature**. A fever may suggest meningitis or encephalitis

Table 5.10 Doses of benzodiazepines for termination of seizures

Child has IV or IO access	Child has no access
Lorazepam (IV or IO) 0.1 mg/kg Max dose 4mg	Midazolam (buccal) 0.5 mg/kg *or* Diazepam (rectal) 0.5 mg/kg

IM, intramuscular; IV, intravenous.

as an underlying cause or overdose with ecstasy, cocaine or salicylates.

– **Look for rashes and bruises**. Purpura may be indicative of meningococcal septicaemia or be a result of non-accidental injury (with head injury as the possible cause for the seizures).

Further management

■ **Assess and treat underlying cause**. It is important to identify, through the history and through clinical signs, what might be the underlying cause for the seizure. *Do not perform a lumbar puncture in a child who is unconscious in case they have raised intracranial pressure*. Consider the following diagnoses, send for appropriate tests and initiate treatment.

– **Hypoglycaemia**. Test for blood glucose levels and treat hypoglycaemia as mentioned above.

– **Hyponatraemia**. A blood sodium level of <130 mmol/L or <135 mmol/L in a child who is still fitting should be corrected with 3 mL/kg of intravenous 3% saline, given over 15 min.

– **Other electrolyte abnormality**. Send bloods for urea, electrolytes, calcium and magnesium and correct any abnormalities.

– **Meningitis or encephalitis**. Ask about history of headache, fever, lethargy, photophobia or irritability. Check temperature and for evidence of neck stiffness or a bulging fontanelle. Treat with cefotaxime 50 mg/kg intravenously and add erythromycin (particularly if history of preceding respiratory illness) and aciclovir (particularly if history of infection with herpes simplex virus) if you suspect encephalitis.

– **Inborn error of metabolism**. If a baby is presenting with seizures, check ammonia levels to identify possible inborn errors of metabolism as the underlying cause.

– **Raised intracranial pressure**. If the child has a history of postural headaches, vomiting or head injury, consider underlying diagnosis of space-occupying lesion or traumatic brain injury leading to raised intracranial pressure which has caused the child to fit. If this is suspected, perform a computed tomography (CT) head scan and arrange transfer to a specialist neurological centre if necessary. *Late signs of raised intracranial pressure such as bradycardia, hypertension and Cheyne–Stokes breathing are pre-terminal signs and must be dealt with immediately with help from senior colleagues prior to proceeding with brain imaging*.

Poisoning

Poisoning may be due to accidental ingestion (usually by a young child) or deliberate overdose (usually by a teenager). Any deliberate overdose should be taken seriously, even if the quantities taken are not likely to be clinically significant, and a mental health and risk assessment performed. *For more information on the psychosocial aspects of deliberate overdose see Chapter 8 – Teenagers.*

Very occasionally, poisoning may be deliberately inflicted by the child's parents or carers but will not present with this history. This is a form of child abuse and has a high associated mortality risk (*see Chapter 4 – Child Protection and Safeguarding for more information about fabricated and induced illness*).

History

Ask about:

■ what has been taken?

■ have they brought the packaging with them?

■ how much has been taken?

■ when was it taken?

■ were multiple different substances taken at multiple different times?

■ is this the first time this has happened?

Symptoms and signs

These will vary depending on the substance or combination of substances that have been taken. *See Table 5.11 for details of common examples.*

Immediate management

■ **Airway**

– **Assess airway** patency. Take measures to open the airway (including airway manoeuvres and the use of airway adjuncts if necessary) and commence Basic Life Support if the child is showing no signs of life.

■ **Breathing**

– **Assess breathing** as detailed in the ABCDE approach above. Check respiratory rate and oxygen saturation levels, look for any signs of respiratory distress and listen for breath sounds and any added sounds.

– **Give high-flow oxygen** if the child has any respiratory abnormalities or decreased consciousness.

– **Ventilate with a bag-valve-mask if necessary**. Several drugs can cause respiratory depression if taken in overdose. Giving oxygen is not sufficient if the child's respiratory rate is low as the saturations may be normal but they will develop hypercapnia as a result of insufficient ventilation. If the child has a low respiratory rate, start ventilation using a bag-valve-mask as detailed in the Advanced Life Support section.

■ **Circulation**

– **Assess circulation** as detailed in the ABCDE approach section above. Check heart rate and rhythm, pulse volume, CAPILLARY REFILL TIME, blood pressure and skin temperature.

– **Perform an ECG** if the heart rate is abnormal or in an irregular rhythm as several substances can cause changes to the ECG and predispose to cardiac arrhythmias.

– **Gain access** either intravenously or intraosseously and take off blood to send to the laboratory. There are some specific blood tests that will be needed for some substances (see Table 5.11). If the substance taken is unknown, send blood for glucose, paracetamol and salicylate levels and toxicology screen.

■ **Disability**

– **Assess neurological status and pupil size**. Depression of conscious level and alteration of pupil size can result from overdose of several different substances. Treat any seizures with benzodiazepines as outlined in the Seizures section.

– **Discuss with a poisons centre**. In all cases of serious poisoning you should discuss the case with a specialist poisons centre for information on specific management. In the UK the National Poisons Information Service has a helpline for specialist advice (0844 892 0111 in the UK, (01) 809 2566 in Ireland). The associated website (www.toxbase.org) has a wealth of useful information on the identification, investigation and management of poisoning and is free to access for all NHS services (find out your department's username and password).

Further management

■ **Test for and correct any acid–base or electrolyte disturbances**.

■ **Consider giving activated charcoal**. Activated charcoal can prevent absorption of some substances if given soon, preferably within 1 h of a substance having been taken. It should only be given if the child is fully conscious (and therefore able to protect their own airway) or if they are intubated and it is given via nasogastric tube.

■ **Gastric lavage in not usually helpful**. Although this was previously quite common, it is now used much less frequently. Discuss with the National Poisons Information Service if you are unsure if this is needed.

Table 5.11 Clinical features, investigation and management of common substances taken in overdose

Substance	Symptoms and signs	Specific investigations	Treatment/ antidote
Paracetamol	None initially; fulminant liver failure can develop over time	Clotting function Albumin Liver function tests Paracetamol level at 4 h after ingestion	Oral charcoal N-acetylcysteine
Salicylates	Tachypnoea Fever Mixed metabolic acidosis and respiratory alkalosis Enlarged anion gap (>18)	pH Chloride Bicarbonate Sodium Potassium Salicylate levels initially at 2 h and then repeated every 2 h	Oral charcoal Alkalinisation to improve excretion; 1 mmol/kg of sodium bicarbonate infused over 4 h
Opiates (including methaodone)	Low respiratory rate Hypotension Small pupils Reduced consciousness	Opiate levels	Naloxone 10 micrograms/kg IV (maximum of 2 mg in one dose). May need repeated doses of naloxone as its half-life is much shorter than that of opiates. Normalise carbon dioxide before giving naloxone or it can cause arrhythmias
Tricyclic antidepressants	Hypotension Seizures Large pupils Metabolic acidosis Cardiac arrhythmias Tachycardia Sinus bradycardia (preterminal sign)	pH Chloride Bicarbonate Sodium Potassium ECG	Alkalinisation to an arterial pH of 7.45–7.5 reduces the toxic effects on the heart. Hyperventilation and sodium bicarbonate infusion can be used to achieve this

(Continued)

Table 5.11 (cont'd)

Substance	Symptoms and signs	Specific investigations	Treatment/ antidote
Iron	Shock Gastrointestinal bleeding Vomiting Diarrhoea Abdominal pain Drowsiness Seizures Enlarged anion gap Metabolic acidosis Hyperglycaemia	pH Chloride Bicarbonate Sodium Potassium Glucose	Gastric lavage and sometimes whole-bowel irrigation may be indicated in large overdoses (>20 mg/ kg). Discuss with poisons centre. Desferrioxamine infusion
Cocaine	Tachycardia Cardiac arrhythmias Hypertension Large pupils Fever Chest pain (as a result of coronary artery spasm)	Troponin ECG	Benzodiazepines, aspirin and high-flow oxygen can be given for acute coronary syndrome. Discuss with the poisons centre
Ecstasy	Cardiac arrhythmias Hyperthermia Metabolic acidosis Increased muscle tone Agitation Anxiety Tachycardia Hyperreflexia Visual disturbances	pH ECG	Activated charcoal Diazepam for anxiety Active cooling if temperature >39°C
Alcohol (ethanol)	Low respiratory rate Metabolic acidosis Enlarged anion gap Hypothermia Hypoglycaemia	pH Chloride Bicarbonate Sodium Potassium Glucose	Correct hypoglycaemia

ECG, electrocardiogram; IV, intravenous.

Diabetic ketoacidosis

Children with diabetic ketoacidosis (DKA) could already have known diabetes or be presenting for the first time before a diagnosis has been made. Careful monitoring and treatment are needed as children can die from DKA, usually as a result of cerebral oedema, hypokalaemia or aspiration pneumonia. Children can appear deceptively well despite very poor blood results; always involve senior colleagues in the initial assessment and management of children with DKA and consider transfer to a paediatric intensive care unit if necessary (particularly for children under 2 years, those with a pH <7.1, reduced consciousness or signs of shock).

History

Ask about:

- polyuria
- polydypsia
- blurred vision
- unusual smelling breath (some people say smells like fruit or pear drops)
- weight loss
- compliance with insulin if already diagnosed with diabetes
- preceding illness.

Symptoms

- Abdominal pain
- Vomiting
- Drowsiness
- Fever (evidence of concurrent illness which may have precipitated ketoacidosis)

Signs

- Dehydrated
- Hyperglycaemia >11 mmol/L
- pH <7.3
- Bicarbonate <15 mmol/L
- Blood ketones >3 mmol/L
- Drowsiness
- Tachypnoea (Kussmaul respiration)
- Breath smells of ketones
- Glucose and ketones in urine

Immediate management

- **Airway**
- **– Assess and maintain patent airway**.
- **– Consider nasogastric tube insertion** to drain stomach contents if the child is vomiting or has reduced conscious levels.
- **Breathing**
- **– Give high-flow oxygen** at 15 L/min via a non-rebreathe mask.
- **Circulation**
- **– Gain access**, ideally with two intravenous cannulae, but if you are struggling to gain access use the intraosseous route in a child who is acutely unwell. Take off blood for full blood count, BLOOD GAS, urea and electrolytes, creatinine, calcium, albumin, glucose and ketones. Also send blood for salicylate levels if overdose is a possibility as poisoning with salicylates can mimic DKA.

Table 5.12 Degree of dehydration

Percentage	Remarks
Mild 3%	Only just clinically detectable
Moderate 5%	Dry mucous membranes, reduced skin turgor
Severe 8%	Above with sunken eyes
Shocked	Rapid thready pulse, tachycardia, +/− hypotension. **Do not use capillary refill time to determine shock as this is not accurate in diabetic ketoacidosis**

Adapted from BSPED guidelines.

– **Assess level of dehydration** and record your findings in the notes. This is useful for comparison later on and is important to assess carefully to guide fluid replacement volumes. The child's percentage dehydration needs to be assessed based on clinical signs (see Table 5.12) because actual weight loss is not helpful in this instance given that weight loss is a presenting feature of diabetes.

– **Treat shock** with slow fluid boluses of 10 mL/kg of normal saline and reassess carefully before giving repeat boluses (up to a maximum of 30 mL/kg if child remains shocked). Do not overestimate or treat shock too aggressively with fluids. Keep a record of exactly how much fluid is given as boluses as this should be removed from the ongoing fluid needs as cerebral oedema is a significant risk with overly rapid rehydration in DKA.

■ **Disability**

– **Assess and record conscious level**. This is important to assess and document regularly in order to monitor carefully for any change that may indicate developing cerebral oedema.

– **Monitor for signs of cerebral oedema**. In addition to altered conscious level, children with cerebral oedema may develop headache and irritability, altered papillary responses, bradycardia and hypertension. **If you suspect cerebral oedema, discuss immediately with senior colleagues and local critical care transfer team to arrange transport to an intensive care unit.**

Further management

■ **Rehydrate over 48 h**. Children presenting in DKA can be profoundly dehydrated, but rapid rehydration has been found to increase the risk of the child developing cerebral oedema (a potentially fatal complication of DKA). Children who are less than 5% dehydrated, have only mild acidosis and are not vomiting may be suitable for oral rehydration rather than intravenous fluids (British Society of Paediatric Endocrinology and Diabetes 2009). For children who require intravenous fluids, do the following.

– **Use altered maintenance fluid values**. Normal maintenance fluid calculations give too large a volume for use in DKA, so instead use the values given in Table 5.13.

– **Calculate replacement fluid requirements** based on your assessment of percentage dehydration as detailed above. ***Overestimating the degree of dehydration is dangerous as overcorrection with fluids can cause cerebral oedema. Do not use more than 8% dehydration in replacement fluid calculations and give the replacement volume over 48 h.*** *For details of how to calculate replacement fluid treatment, see Chapter 7 – Prescribing in Children, or use this formula:*

Table 5.13 Maintenance fluid values to be used in children with DKA

Weight (kg)	Rate (mL/kg/24 h)
<13	80
13–20	65
20–35	55
35–60	45
>60	35

Adapted from BSPED Guidelines.

Children who are less than 5% dehydrated, have only mild acidosis and are not vomiting may be suitable for subcutaneous insulin rather than requiring a continuous intravenous insulin infusion.

$$\text{Deficit (mL)} = \% \text{ dehydration} \times \text{body weight (kg)} \times 10$$

– **Subtract the volume of any fluid boluses given from the total**. If the child was shocked and fluid boluses were given on admission, these need to be subtracted from the total volume infused over 48 h.

■ **Monitor ketones and pH**. Insulin should be given even after normal blood glucose levels are achieved as it is needed to switch off ketogenesis and allow

$$\text{Fluids for 48h} = (2 \times \text{maintenance value (from Table 5.13)} + \text{deficit volume}) - \text{fluid boluses}$$

$$\text{Hourly rate} = \frac{(48\text{h maintenance} + \text{deficit volume}) - \text{fluid boluses given}}{48}$$

– **Use the correct type of fluid**. Start by giving 0.9% saline for at least 12 h, then change to 0.9% saline with 5% glucose once blood glucose <14 mmol/L. **Add 20 mmol of potassium chloride to each 500 mL bag of fluids given**.

■ **Replace insulin**. Insulin treatment should not be started until fluids have been running for 1 h as there is some evidence that this reduces the risk of cerebral oedema. Start intravenous insulin at a constant rate of 0.1 unit/kg/h.

resolution of the acidosis. This means that you should continue giving insulin at the same rate and add dextrose to the fluids in order to maintain normal blood glucose levels. Keep insulin at a steady infusion until pH is >7.3 when rate can be reduced to 0.05 unit/kg/h. If the child's blood glucose levels are reducing at a rate of more than 5 mmol/h, the insulin infusion rate can be reduced temporarily or fluid changed to 0.9% saline with 10% glucose after consultation with senior colleagues.

Treat hypoglycaemia. If blood glucose falls to less than 4 mmol/L, give 2 mL/kg of 10% dextrose and discuss with a consultant the possibility of increased concentration of glucose in the intravenous fluids.

Monitor potassium. Potassium should be replaced as a matter of course (add 20 mmol to every 500 mL of fluid infused) because although the initial serum potassium may be high, the total body potassium is likely to be low. Initiation of insulin drives potassium back into the cells, which can result in a dangerously low blood potassium level unless corrected.

Look for and treat any underlying illness. Development of DKA may have resulted from the child having an underlying illness. Perform a detailed history and examination, followed by relevant investigations (such as a chest x-ray, urinalysis and blood cultures) to look for evidence of underlying infection, which should be treated if necessary.

Trauma

The same principles of the structured ABCDE approach apply to a child who has suffered an injury but with a few minor additions. The majority of serious trauma cases will be called ahead by the ambulance crew, giving you time to assemble a trauma team (which should include orthopaedics and general surgeons in addition to the normal resuscitation team). However, in some cases (for example, in cases of stabbings) the child may present to the department independently and you will receive no warning. In these instances, put out a trauma call immediately to summon all the relevant people (it is far better to send them all away again if not needed than to have insufficient support and risk compromising the quality of care you can provide).

Catastrophic external haemorrhage

It is rare that external bleeding will be significant enough to warrant deviation from the usual ABCDE approach and minor bleeding injuries should only be dealt with after initial resuscitation has taken place. However, in situations where haemorrhage is extreme and will be rapidly fatal unless dealt with, this warrants immediate management. *Apply direct pressure to the wound and ask someone to put out a trauma call (2222) if your surgical colleagues are not already present or call the emergency services (999) if you are in the community*. Tourniquets can be applied in the case of severe limb injuries causing catastrophic bleeding.

Airway and cervical spine control

Assessment and management of the airway are the same as for the unwell child except for the following.

Use a jaw thrust to open the airway and avoid a head tilt in case of possible cervical spine injury.

Clear the mouth. Perform suction with a Yankauer suction catheter or remove foreign bodies with Magill's forceps (see Fig. 5.17) to remove vomit, blood or foreign bodies from the mouth but only as far as you can see. **Do not put the tip of the forceps or Yankauer further down than you can see**.

■ **Stabilise the cervical spine**, using your hands to support either side of the head to encourage them not to move their neck. Do not force this but try to calmly reassure the child and enlist the help of the parents if necessary as the child struggling against you can make matters worse. Put a neck collar on the child until the cervical spine has been imaged and x-rays cleared if they are able to tolerate it. If not, you may have to designate one member of the team to providing ongoing manual stabilisation (this will also allow for much easier intubation if needed as collars can impede sufficient opening of the jaw).

■ **Protect the airway from vomit**. If a child is vomiting but is still required to lie flat on their back in order to protect the spine then this can cause potential problems for maintaining the airway. If the child vomits, tilt the trolley head down so that the vomit pools in the roof of the mouth rather than going down the trachea and use suction to remove it.

Breathing

The same principles apply as for with the ABCDE approach outlined above but there are some additional diagnoses that require immediate management. Most of these will require management with advanced practical procedures (such as insertion of a chest drain or intubation) that can only be performed by senior colleagues with

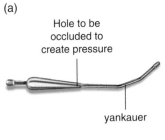

(a)

Hole to be occluded to create pressure

yankauer

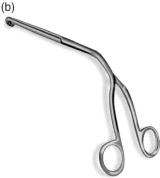

(b)

Figure 5.17 (a) Yankauer sucker; (b) Macgill's forceps.

experience of doing so. The following measures can be undertaken by you whilst awaiting assistance.

■ **Put on high-flow oxygen** for all children with trauma. Give 15 L/min via a non-rebreathe mask.

■ **Tension pneumothorax**. This can occur occasionally without a history of trauma but happens much more commonly following trauma and you should have a high index of suspicion and make the diagnosis **clinically** (do not waste time ordering a chest x-ray as by then it may be too late). Signs suggestive of a tension pneumothorax include:

– reduced chest movement and reduced breath sounds on the side of the pneumothorax

– hyperresonance to percussion on the side of the pneumothorax

– distended neck veins

– shock and hypoxia

– trachea deviated away from the side of the pneumothorax.

To decompress, **insert a wide-bore cannula in the midclavicular line in the second intercostal space**. Aim just above the top edge of the third rib (in order to avoid the neurovascular bundle running along the bottom edge of the second rib). You should hear a hissing noise as air is released through the needle. Needle decompression is a temporary emergency measure to relieve a tension pneumothorax but the child will also need insertion of a chest drain to prevent air from accumulating again.

■ **Open pneumothorax**. This can occur after a penetrating injury to the child's chest. Signs suggestive of an open pneumothorax include:

– reduced chest movement and reduced breath sounds on the side of the pneumothorax

– hyperresonance to percussion on the side of the pneumothorax

– sucking and blowing sound as air passes in and out of the wound.

If you find an open pneumothorax, stick an occlusive dressing over the wound and stick it down **on three sides only**. This then acts as a flap valve so that air cannot be sucked into the pleural space through the wound but can still escape to avoid development of a tension pneumothorax.

Circulation with haemorrhage control

Assess circulation as detailed in the ABCDE approach above, including assessment for signs of shock.

■ **Gain access**. Ideally two large-bore intravenous cannulae. If you are having difficulty gaining intravenous access do not waste time but instead try the intraosseous route. *Do not insert intraosseous access into the peripheral portion of a fractured limb*.

■ **Send off blood for cross-match**. Assessment of blood type (ABO typing) can take 10–15 min for urgent cases. Full cross-matching usually takes closer to 45–60 min. Use O-negative or type-specific blood whilst awaiting cross-matched blood.

■ **Give fluid bolus if there are signs of shock**. A fluid bolus of 10 mL/kg of 0.9% saline should be given if the child is showing signs of shock. Do not be too aggressive in your fluid replacement as returning the child's blood pressure to normal may disrupt clots and increase the rate of bleeding.

■ **Reassess and repeat bolus if needed**. Repeat boluses of fluid can be given if necessary. If 40 mL/kg of saline has been given then further volume replacement should be with blood (use O-negative blood if urgent).

■ **Stop the bleeding**. The only way to properly stabilise the child is to stop the bleeding. *This will require urgent input from surgical colleagues, so enlist their help immediately if they are not already present and inform theatres or a critical care transfer team if surgery cannot take place at your unit.*

Disability and assessment of head injury

Brain injury can be primary (damage which occurs as a result of direct impact) and secondary (further damage as a result of hypoxia, hypotension and raised intracranial pressure). The key aim of immediate management in children with head injury is to minimise the amount of secondary injury that occurs.

As soon as serious head injury is suspected, order an urgent CT head scan and contact your nearest critical care transfer service or neurosurgical team. You will need to assess the child's Glasgow Coma Scale prior to discussion with the neurosurgical team (see Table 5.4 for age-specific Glasgow Coma Scoring).

■ **ABC management** as above, if completed properly, should help to minimise hypoxia and hypotension. Early infusion of blood products if needed can minimise dilutional anaemia.

■ **DEFG: Don't Ever Forget Glucose**. Test blood glucose and treat any detected hypoglycaemia or hyperglycaemia.

■ **Perform an emergency CT head scan if indicated**. Specific indications for emergency CT head scan are outlined in NICE guidelines on head injury available at www.nice.org.uk.

Critical care transfer services

Children who are very unwell may need to be transferred to a specialist centre with a paediatric intensive care unit or to a unit which is able to provide specific treatments such as neurosurgery or cardiac specialist therapy. There are many different specialist critical care transfer teams, detailed below, usually run by paediatric intensive care or paediatric anaesthetic consultants. They are able to transfer very unwell children safely to a place where they can receive specialist care and many of them will also provide advice over the phone about the management of sick children and help to locate a paediatric intensive care bed. Some of the websites also have useful emergency clinical guidelines and drug calculators for commonly used medications. If your regional transport team is unable to provide transfer to an appropriate unit it may forward your call on to another service. These numbers and services may change over time; for an up-to-date list visit the Paediatric Intensive Care Society website (www.ukpics.org.uk).

North West England

North West and North Wales Paediatric Transport Service (NWTS)
Region: North West England and North Wales
Based at: Royal Manchester Children's Hospital and Alder Hey Children's Hospital

Referrals and advice hotline: 08000 84 83 82

Website: www.nwts.nhs.uk

Clinical guidelines available on website: some

North East England

Yorkshire and Humber Infant and Children's Transport Service (Embrace)

Region: Yorkshire and Humber

Based at: Sheffield Children's NHS Foundation Trust

Referrals number: 0845 147 2472

General enquiries: 0114 305 3005

Website: http://www.sheffieldchildrens.nhs.uk/embrace

Clinical guidelines available on website: yes

West Midlands

Kids Intensive Care and Decision Support (KIDS)

Region: West Midlands

Based at: Birmingham Children's Hospital and University Hospital of North Staffordshire

Referrals and advice hotline: 0300 200 1100

Website: www.kids.bch.nhs.uk

Clinical guidelines available on website: yes

East Midlands

Paediatric and Infant Critical Care Transport Service (PICCTS)

Region: Leicester

Based at: Glenfield Hospital and Leicester Royal Infirmary

Referrals and advice hotline: 0300 300 0023

Website: www.piccts.co.uk

Clinical guidelines available on website: not currently, planned in future

South East England and London

Children's Acute Transport Service (CATS)

Region: North London and South East England

Based at: Great Ormond Street Hospital, St Mary's Hospital and Royal Brompton Hospital

Referrals and advice hotline: 0800 085 0003

Website: www.cats.nhs.uk

Clinical guidelines available on website: yes

South Thames Retrieval Service

Region: South London and South East England

Based at: Evelina Children's Hospital and St Thomas' Hospital

Referrals and advice hotline: 020 7188 5000

Website: www.strs.nhs.uk

Clinical guidelines available on website: yes

South Central and South West England

Southampton Oxford Retrieval Team (SORT)

Region: South England

Based at: Southampton General Hospital and John Radcliffe Hospital, Oxford

Referrals and advice hotline: 023 8077 5502

Website: www.sort.nhs.uk

Clinical guidelines available on website: Yes

North Wales

North West and North Wales Paediatric Transport Service (NWTS)

Region: North West England and North Wales

Based at: Royal Manchester Children's Hospital and Alder Hey Children's Hospital

Referrals and advice hotline: 08000 84 83 82

Website: www.nwts.nhs.uk

Clinical guidelines available on website: some

East Scotland

Scottish National Paediatric Retrieval Service

Region: East Scotland

Based at: Royal Hospital for Sick Children Edinburgh

Referrals and advice hotline: 0131 536 0919

Website: www.snprs.scot.nhs.uk

Clinical guidelines available on website: yes

West Scotland

Scottish National Paediatric Retrieval Service

Region: West Scotland

Based at: Royal Hospital for Sick Children Glasgow (Yorkhill)

Referrals and advice hotline: 0141 201 6923

Website: www.snprs.scot.nhs.uk

Clinical guidelines available on website: drug information and procedures only

Northern Ireland

Child or Neonate Needing Emergency Critical Care Transport (CONNECCT)

Region: Northern Ireland

Based at: Royal Belfast Hospital for Sick Children

Referrals and advice hotline: 02890 632449

Website: no website currently available

Useful websites

British Thoracic Society: www.brit-thoracic.org.uk. Has nationally approved guidance on the management of acute and chronic asthma.

Resuscitation Council: www.resus.org.uk. The latest paediatric and neonatal Basic Life Support and Advanced Life Support guidelines and a reference chart for emergency drug doses are available to download free of charge.

National Institute for Health and Clinical Excellence (NICE): www.nice.org.uk. Has various guidelines relating to topics such as fever, head injury and diarrhoea and vomiting.

Paediatric Intensive Care Society: www.ukpics.org.uk. Has a page containing details of regional critical care transport services.

Children's Acute Transport Service (CATS): www.cats.nhs.uk. Has lots of diagnosis-specific emergency guidelines on the website and an electronic drug calculator that automatically calculates doses of many commonly used drugs if you enter the child's weight and date of birth.

TOXBASE: www.toxbase.org. An online database of information about identification, investigation and management of poisoning.

References

Advanced Life Support Group (2011) *Advanced Paediatric Life Support*. Wiley-Blackwell, Oxford.

British Society of Paediatric Endocrinology and Diabetes (2009) *BSPED Recommended DKA Guidelines 2009*. British Society of Paediatric Endocrinology and Diabetes, Bristol.

Chapter 6
PRACTICAL PROCEDURES

A lot of people find it very daunting at first when learning to perform procedures on children. You will already have learnt lots of the relevant skills from doing some of the same procedures in adult medicine but some procedures (such as capillary blood gas sampling) will not be familiar.

Setting up

Having the right environment for performing procedures is really important and is quite different from the adult medicine approach. Most paediatric wards will have a treatment room where procedures are normally carried out rather than doing them at the bedside. Having a separate room helps you to have more space and a more controlled environment and means that other children on the ward aren't upset by hearing another child in distress. It is also an important message to the child that their bed is a safe place where nasty things like procedures don't happen.

Details about specific procedures are covered below, but these general principles apply to all procedures in children.

■ **Prepare your equipment**. It is important to set up all your equipment beforehand so that it is ready to grab when you are in the middle of a procedure – with young children you will have to act quickly as even with help, it is difficult to keep them still for long and you don't want to prolong their distress.

■ **Prepare pain relief**. The specifics of what to use will vary between the different procedures but it is always important to consider how you plan to minimise pain and allow plenty of time for topical agents to have an effect.

■ **Prepare the child and the parents**. It is important to talk the child and their parents through what will happen and why it is necessary to perform the procedure. Explain to the child in simple terms that they are able to understand. Don't tell them that it will not hurt if this is not true as you will lose their trust. Talking them through what to expect will make the whole experience less frightening. Take the opportunity to ask the parents what they think will work best for their child in terms of distracting them or helping them to cope.

■ **Involve a play specialist**. Play specialist are experts in child development and age-appropriate play. They are

The Hands-on Guide to Practical Paediatrics, First Edition. Rebecca Hewitson and Caroline Fertleman.
© 2014 John Wiley & Sons, Ltd. Published 2014 by John Wiley & Sons, Ltd.
Companion Website: www.wileyhandsonguides.com/paediatrics

fantastic at engaging children in play in order to distract them from what is happening with the procedure and can make the whole thing go much more smoothly. If they are not available then medical students can often be very good at providing distraction by playing games or blowing bubbles.

■ **Position the child appropriately**. Setting up the room, your equipment and the child in the best position can really increase your chances of success. Make sure that you have positioned the child in a way which means you can comfortably perform the procedure. This will vary between procedures and specifics are advised for each below.

■ **Prepare yourself**. Make sure that you wash your hands thoroughly before starting the procedure. Wear gloves and an apron (blood can splash everywhere with a toddler thrashing around) to protect yourself and your clothes and bear in mind that some procedures should be done in sterile conditions (with sterile gown, gloves and drapes). Use the smallest pair of gloves you can fit into so that they are tight around your fingertips as this really helps with dexterity. If the procedure is going to take a while to perform, sit down at the same height as child so that you are comfortable and can keep a steady hand.

■ **Praise the child afterwards**. Make sure that you praise the child afterwards for tolerating the procedure. Rewards such as certificates or stickers can also be much appreciated. Remember that the parents may also be feeling quite stressed by the procedure and a kind word to them wouldn't go amiss either.

Cannulation

For a checklist of equipment which you need for putting in a cannula see Box 6.1.

Cannulation in children and NEO-NATES takes time and practice to get the hang of but most of the principles of insertion are the same as for adults. However, there are some differences (even in the equipment you will need) so consider the following before attempting to cannulate a child.

■ **Prepare your equipment**. This includes taking the lids of bottles if you plan to drip blood into MICROTAINERS, flushing the extension set with saline and opening all the packets containing your equipment (you should either put your equipment in a sterile tray or place it back inside the open packets to protect them).

■ **Choose the correct cannula size**. Look at the child's veins before putting on the anaesthetic cream to get an idea of how big they are. The veins can be much more difficult to see properly after the anaesthetic cream as the skins swells and can become erythematous. You also need to consider what will be given through the cannula and how quickly (obviously, the bigger the cannula, the more quickly you can deliver fluids and don't forget that there is a big change in maximum flow rates with a small change in cannula diameter). The larger the gauge number, the smaller the cannula is. *See Table 6.1 for details of which cannula size to use.*

■ **Choose the correct site**. The back of the hand tends to be the best position for a cannula in young children and you

Box 6.1 Checklist of equipment needed for cannula insertion

■ Gloves

■ Sterile alcohol skin wipes

■ Cannulas (take a few of different sizes with you)

■ A sticky cannula dressing

■ An extension set (sometimes referred to as a T-piece or octopus)

■ A syringe

■ A vial of sterile 0.9% saline for injection

■ Gauze

■ Sharps bin

Extras sometimes needed

■ A bung (needed for the end of some types of extension sets)

■ A tourniquet (for older children)

■ A splint (for younger children in order to immobilise the hand you have cannulated)

■ A bandage (for younger children to ensure the cannula is well secured and to hold the splint on)

■ An extra syringe for drawing blood

■ Blood bottles or mircotainers

■ Capillary tube (for blood gas or SBR)

■ Culture bottle, extra alcohol wipes for the bottle top, sterile needle for transfer of blood into the culture bottle

Table 6.1 Different sizes of cannula and their uses.

Gauge	Colour (this may vary, check the gauge size)	Child's age
24 G or 'Neoflon'	Yellow	Any child under 2
22 G	Blue	Toddlers or any age of child with small veins
20 G	Pink	Older children with larger veins or those needing resuscitation
18 G	Green	Teenagers requiring rapid resuscitation

can also use veins on the top of the feet in babies. In older children, you may be able to site a cannula in the antecubital fossa but these larger veins may be best left for emergency situations when access is really needed (for younger children, they should be avoided for routine use as the cannula is likely to become dislodged by the child bending and straightening their arm). If you really need venous access in a child who is peripherally shut down then the long saphenous vein can be a useful site. It runs just anterior to the medial malleolus. The scalp can also sometimes be a good site in babies, but this can look rather alarming for parents and needs to be explained.

■ **Prepare pain relief**. Make sure that the child has had anaesthetic cream on the area you plan to cannulate for at least 40 min for Ametop gel or 60 min for EMLA cream before attempting the procedure. This can help to numb the skin and make the whole process much less painful for the child. If not left on for sufficient time then these topical preparations will not work properly. Obviously, if the child is unwell and in urgent need of intravenous access for medications or fluid resuscitation, you would not be able to wait this long and would have to cannulate in the absence of analgesia. Some older children may prefer to have a cold spray (ethyl chloride) sprayed on immediately before insertion of a cannula to numb the skin instead of anaesthetic cream. For babies, sucrose is sometimes used as an analgesic although there is some evidence that suckling with or without

sucrose (such as on a dummy or a gloved finger) may be equally effective.

■ **Get someone else to help you**. It is essential to have an extra pair of hands in addition to the play specialist and the child's parent to help you hold the child still and pass you equipment. Having someone who is experienced at doing this can make an enormous difference to your chances of success as they will be better at holding the child's arm still and can anticipate the steps in the process. *Don't* use a parent to hold the child's arm still as they will probably not feel comfortable holding on firmly enough to restrain them and you will end up with a moving target.

■ **Position the child appropriately**. For younger children it can be useful to put the child on their parent's lap so that they are sitting face to face. You can then bring the child's arm underneath the parent's arm and distract them by positioning the play specialist on the opposite side. Make sure that they are positioned so that you can comfortably reach them (probably with you kneeling down) as if you are uncomfortable or in an awkward position it will be much more difficult to keep a steady hand. *See Video 3 for more details.*

■ **Hold the skin taut**. Tethering the vein by holding the overlying skin taut will straighten out any tortuous veins and help to stop them skipping out of the way of your needle.

■ **Collecting blood from a cannula**. If you are likely to need blood samples, it is ideal to take blood at the same time as the cannula is inserted to avoid the child having to endure a separate needle for taking bloods. In older children, you may be able to use a syringe or vacutainer blood bottles to draw back blood from the cannula just after you have inserted it (and before flushing!). However, in younger children and babies, their small veins may collapse under the pressure applied by the suction of the syringe. In this case it is best to let blood drip from the end of the cannula into the paediatric blood bottles before you apply the extension set.

And don't forget the general rules mentioned above.

- Prepare the child and parents.
- Involve a play specialist.
- Prepare yourself.
- Praise the child afterwards.

Taking blood (including heel prick sampling)

For older children, taking blood can be done in the same way as in adults (apart from remembering to use analgesia and distraction techniques) and you can use normal adult bottles. However, for smaller children you may need to use a different technique for taking blood and collect the samples in paediatric sized tubes (sometimes called MICROTAINERS) which only need less than a millilitre of blood to fill them.

Heel prick sampling

For a checklist of equipment needed for a heel prick sample, see Box 6.2.

HEEL PRICK sampling can be a useful way of collecting blood from babies and toddlers. Basically, this technique relies on you catching drips of blood into the

Box 6.2   Checklist of equipment needed for capillary blood gas sample and/or other heel prick samples

■ Sterile alcohol skin wipes

■ A plaster or dressing (for afterwards)

■ Petroleum jelly

■ Spring-loaded lancets (take 2–3 with you)

■ Gloves

■ Gauze

■ Capillary tubes and bungs for the ends (if taking capillary blood gas sample or for an SBR in some units)

■ Paediatric blood bottles for other blood needed from a heel prick sample

blood tubes. This can be quite challenging at first but as the tubes are so tiny, you don't need many drops before they are adequately filled. The process of squeezing blood from the capillary bed can cause haemolysis of the sample so it may sometimes be better to attempt venepuncture even in babies (details below). Here are some suggestions to increase your chances of successfully taking a heel prick sample.

■ **Prepare your equipment**. Take the lids off any paediatric blood bottles you are using and any safety caps off the lancets. Put some gauze or an absorbent pad on the floor or the parent's lap or in the cot (depending on how the baby is positioned) to catch any stray drips.

■ **Prepare pain relief**. Traditionally a tiny dose of oral sucrose (from a syringe or on a dummy) is given to babies just before painful procedures as it is thought to reduce their response to pain. Breastfeeding or breast milk from a syringe appears to be just as effective for analgesia and some units have moved towards this as an alternative to products like Sweet-Ease (Shah et al. 2012).

■ **Prepare the child and parents**. You will mostly be performing heel pricks on babies who will not be able to understand what is happening but you can try explaining very simply to toddlers. It helps to explain to the parents what you are doing and why. It may also be useful to warn them that often the bit which babies are most distressed by is restraining the movement of their leg, not the pain caused by lancing the skin.

■ **Position the child appropriately**. For babies and toddlers this can be best with the child lying on the parent's lap. Having their feet hanging slightly downwards will allow gravity to help with collecting the sample. Most people use their non-dominant hand for squeezing and dominant hand for scraping the blood drops into the tube but find which way round is best for you and position the child accordingly.

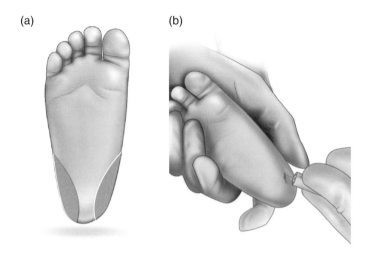

(a)   (b)

Figure 6.1 Where on the foot to take a heel prick sample (a) and how to hold the foot (b).

■ **Choose the correct site**. Chosing the correct place to use your lancet is important to maximise your chances of success and minimise the pain it causes. Make sure that you go for the fleshy part on the side of the heel as this is rich in capillary supply and will bleed well. Try to avoid using the sole of the foot if possible as this is much more painful. *See Fig. 6.1 for the correct sites for heel prick samples.*

■ **Make sure that the baby's feet are warm**. If the baby has cold feet this will make collecting the sample difficult as cold feet are the result of capillary constriction, meaning that you won't get much blood out. Try putting socks on and asking the parent to sit holding their child's feet to warm them up for a few minutes first.

■ **Catching the drips**. The hard part can be managing to catch each drop of blood in the bottle. The blood doesn't usually drip from the foot but clings to it in a blob on the surface of the skin. This means that you need to scrape it off the skin and into the tube using the rim of the tube. This can be very tricky and end up with you smearing blood everywhere and very little actually getting into the bottle. Being deliberate and rapid in the way you collect the drops can help, as can spreading a very thin layer of petroleum jelly on the skin to help encourage the blood to remain in distinct droplets. If things are getting messy, wipe the skin with some sterile gauze as this will help further drops of blood to form in distinct droplets again.

■ **Holding the foot**. Hold the foot dorsiflexed and squeeze around the ankle and the sole of the foot (with your fingers and thumb respectively). The technique of squeezing in order to get the best blood flow takes practice. *Watch Video 3 for details and see Fig. 6.1 for how to hold the foot.*

■ **Let go between squeezes**. Don't just continually squeeze the baby's foot in the desperate hope that it will keep bleeding as this doesn't work. You need to release all pressure on the foot every couple of seconds in order to allow the capillaries to refill with blood.

■ **If you are taking more than one bottle, use more than one lancet**. If you need to fill more than one paediatric bottle, it is unlikely that you will be able to collect all the blood from one lance. It can be kinder to start out by doing two lances just next to one another which will enable you to collect sufficient blood much more quickly rather than spending a long time squeezing the foot, upsetting the baby more and possibly also haemolysing the blood sample.

  Top Tip

If you are using MICROTAINERS and need to be able to quickly switch between them whilst collecting blood (from a HEEL PRICK, cannula or venepuncture), take all the lids off first and place them in the inside of a roll of tape in order to hold them upright.

Once you have finished and replaced the lids on the bottles, remember to invert them a few times to mix the blood with the additives in the tube – this can avoid having your sample rejected by the laboratory.

Don't forget to **involve a play specialist** to distract the child if they are old enough to benefit from distraction techniques, while playing music can help to soothe babies.

Venepuncture in babies

The difference with venepuncture in babies compared to older children is the size of the needle you use and the way you collect the blood. In babies, if you tried to use a butterfly needle with a syringe or a vacutainer system to collect blood, the veins would collapse under the pressure. This means that you need to collect blood by allowing it to drip from the end of the needle into the paediatric blood bottles.

■ **Choose the correct kind of needle**. Some units will have special needles designed specifically for taking blood from newborns (they are usually either 23 G or 25 G and have a small flange to hold onto on one side), whilst others will use a butterfly needle or a cannula instead. You may see people using butterfly needles with the tubing cut off or a needle with the hub broken off the end, but this is not considered best practice and could leave you vulnerable medico-legally should anything go wrong as you would have modified the equipment against the manufacturer's advice. Whichever one of these you use, the technique involves allowing blood to drip from the blunt end of the needle into the bottles (or attaching a syringe and very gently withdrawing the plunger if using a butterfly needle). You can occlude the vein between bottles to stop the flow of blood.

■ **Get someone to help you**. Ask someone else to hold the baby's arm still and to act as a tourniquet by squeezing. Squeezing and releasing can help with blood flow but be careful not to dislodge the needle as this can slowly work it out of position. If blood flow stops then try advancing the needle a tiny bit as this may be enough to place the needle back into the vein and blood to flow again.

■ **Anchor the vein**. You should hold the skin taut over the vein in order to anchor it and stop it from moving away from your needle.

■ **Collecting blood cultures**. You cannot use the method of catching drops of blood for collecting blood cultures. Instead, you need to use a closed system (such as a butterfly needle with a syringe) in order to avoid contamination of the sample. You may also sometimes see people using a needle and syringe to draw up blood that has drained into the hub of a cannula or needle (before it drips) but this can lead to contamination of the sample and is not recommended. For paediatric blood cultures, you only need to use one bottle rather than two. The volume of blood needed will depend on the age and weight of the child. For newborns you only need to collect between 1 mL and 1.5 mL of blood for cultures; for older children you will need 3–5 mL of blood. For teenagers whose circulating blood volume is almost equivalent to adults, you may wish to use two culture bottles (one aerobic and one anaerobic) and collect 10–20 mL of blood.

Capillary blood gas

See Box 6.2 for a checklist of equipment needed for a capillary blood gas sample.

This can be quite a tricky technique at first but is pretty straightforward once you get the hang of it. Capillary blood gas sampling involves taking blood from the capillary bed (usually in a child's heel) using a capillary tube which sucks the blood up by capillary action! A capillary tube is a small, see-through straw-shaped tube made of either glass or plastic. Capillary action is

---

 Top Tip

If you just have one small air bubble in the sample, rather than taking a whole new sample it is possible to get rid of the air bubble. Take another, empty capillary tube and put the end against the tube containing your sample. Then tilt the two tubes so that blood flows from the original tube into the empty one and stop (i.e. move the tubes back to being horizontal) when you get to the air bubble. Take the tubes apart and tip the original one very slightly so that the blood goes right to the end of the tube and pushes the air bubble out. Then put the two ends of the tubes together (making sure that there are no air bubbles in either end) and tip all the blood back into one tube. You should now have just one tube of blood with no air bubble in it! *See Video 4 for more details.*

the mechanism which causes liquid to be drawn up into a narrow tube so that when you touch the tube to a drop of blood, it automatically enters the tube.

The difficult bit in this process is avoiding getting any air bubbles in the sample as this means that the machine will reject the sample. The secret of successfully collecting a capillary blood gas sample relies on you holding the tube at the correct angle. If you hold the tube tilted upright too much then the blood doesn't fill the tube (or does so painfully slowly) but if you tilt the tube too far down then you will get air bubbles in your sample.

Make sure that you have had training in how to use the blood gas analysers at your trust as they vary between hospitals. In some units they will have a clot filter on the machine and you can attach your sample directly to this, whilst in others you need to insert a small iron rod into the tube and use a magnet to move it backwards and forwards along the tube to break up any forming clots.

Top Tip

Once you have taken your capillary blood sample, be careful not to spill it everywhere. Some units will have bungs available which you can place on either end of the tube. If not, then keep the tube horizontal whilst transferring it to a gas machine to stop the blood from pouring out of either end.

How to measure a spun bilirubin (SBR)

The equipment used for this will vary between different units (so make sure that you find out the specifics at your hospital) but the general principles in each case are the same.

■ **Collect a sample**. Use the HEEL PRICK technique above to collect a blood sample, making sure that you are using the correct tube to collect the sample. In some trusts, blood for an SBR is collected in special blood bottles, whilst in others it should be collected in a capillary tube.

■ **Spin the sample**. The clue is in the name; a spun bilirubin means that you have to put the blood sample in a centrifuge to spin it. If you are using a capillary tube, you will need to put a small amount of clay into each end of the tube to act as bungs to keep your sample in the tube. The process of spinning the sample separates different components of the blood so that the cells are at the bottom with a layer of plasma on top. The cells appear a dark red colour and the plasma is a translucent yellow colour.

■ **Measure the plasma bilirubin**. A machine called a spectrophotometer is used to shine a light through the plasma component of the sample in order to calculate the amount of bilirubin present. Some machines are designed for slotting in the capillary tube directly (making sure to put the serum layer, not the cell layer, over the light source) but for others you have to transfer some of the serum to a cuvette first. A cuvette is a small container made of either clear plastic or glass which holds the serum as a thin film, allowing a light to be shone through it to measure the bilirubin levels. Use a pipette to draw up a small amount of serum and then inject it into the cuvette before putting the cuvette in the spectrophotometer to measure the bilirubin.

How to measure packed cell volume

This can be done on the same sample used for measuring a spun bilirubin level if you have used a capillary tube to collect the sample. Packed cell volume is exactly as it sounds: you are measuring the size of the layer of cells which have been separated out by spinning the sample in a centrifuge.

You can use a measuring tool (a bit like a ruler) to measure the height of the cell layer which has equivalent values of packed cell volume written on it for you to read off.

Intraosseous access

For a list of equipment needed for gaining intraosseous access, see Box 6.3.

This can be a life-saving procedure in an emergency situation. Bones are very vascular structures so, in resuscitation situations, if it is not possible to get intravenous access you can use intraosseous (IO) access as an alternative method to deliver fluids. If a child is acutely unwell and intravenous access is difficult, don't waste time with multiple attempts at intravenous access; consider gaining IO access instead.

Gaining intraosseous access can be done either manually with an intraosseous needle (sometimes called a Cook needle) or using a mechanical device such as the following.

1 EZ-IO (which is American and therefore pronounced as if saying 'Easy IO') is a device which looks and sounds like a drill. The needles are disposable but

---

Box 6.3   Checklist of equipment needed for gaining intraosseous access

■ Manual needle or mechanical device with correct size needle

■ Sterile gloves

■ Apron

■ 10 mL syringe × 2 (one for saline flush one for collecting bone marrow sample)

■ 20 mL syringe for giving further fluid boluses if needed

■ Alcohol skin wipes or a ChloraPrep sponge

■ Sodium chloride 0.9% for flush

■ Extension set

■ Specimen bottles for sending marrow samples (e.g. for group and save)

■ Tape

the drill device is reusable and battery powered.

2 Bone Injection Gun (BIG) is a spring-loaded device which fires the needle into the intraosseous space. The entire device is disposable.

■ **Preparing the parents**. If you are using an EZ-IO it is worth bearing in mind that this will look incredibly distressing to parents as it looks and sounds like you are drilling into their child's leg (which you sort of are) so try to get someone to distract them or remove them from the room temporarily whilst this happens.

■ **Preparing pain relief**. If you need to gain intraosseous access then the child is probably comatose and you will not have time to delay for analgesia. Insertion of IO needles using the EZ-IO has been done on conscious adults without local anaesthetic and only causes moderate pain but flushing with saline can be very painful in conscious patients (in which case, very slow infusion of 2% lidocaine is recommended before flushing in order to numb the medullary cavity).

■ **Identify the correct site**. There are two main sites commonly used for gaining IO access in children: proximal tibia and distal femur. These sites avoid damaging any growth plates and the proximal tibia is the site most commonly used. The distal tibia is also sometimes used if necessary. *See Fig. 6.2 for sites which can be used for IO access.*

– **Proximal tibia**. Feel for the tibial tuberosity and then move your finger 1–2 cm medially and 2–3 cm peripher-

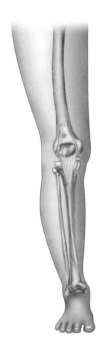

Figure 6.2 *Sites to use for IO access (marked in orange).*

ally. This should put you on the flat surface on the inner aspect of the tibia (see Fig. 6.2).

– **Distal femur**. Feel for the lateral condyle of the femur and then move 3 cm proximally and across to anterior surface in the midline (see Fig. 6.2).

– **Distal tibia**. Feel for the medial mallelous and move 2 cm proximally (this should only be used if you cannot gain access at either of the above suggested sites).

■ **Use the correct size needle**.

– **Manual: 16 G**.

– **EZ-IO:** for children between 3 kg and 40 kg use the pink needle. For children over 40 kg use the blue needle.

– **BIG:** for newborns to children aged 12 years you need to use the red paediatric BIG and turn the red section until the correct age group (and therefore needle depth) for your patient is showing. For children older than 12 years use the blue adult BIG. This has a standard needle depth setting so you do not need to adjust it.

■ **Clean the skin**. Clean the skin over the site with an alcohol wipe or ChloraPrep sponge and allow to dry completely.

■ **Insert the needle**.

– **Manually:** insert the needle through the skin until you feel it touch against bone. With firm downwards pressure (by holding the circular head of the needle in the palm of your hand), use a twisting motion to advance the needle into the bone. You will feel a 'give' as the needle enters the bone marrow cavity, at which point you should immediately stop pushing (to avoid going all the way through the bone and out the other side). Remove the stylet and the needle should remain upright without you holding it if it is in the correct place.

– **EZ-IO:** attach the correct size of needle to the drill handle. Insert the needle through the skin until you feel it touch bone. Once the end of the needle is touching bone, pull the trigger on

the drill to start it. Very little pressure is needed to insert the needle as the drilling action does most of the work (and in fact, if you use too much pressure it won't work as well). Once you feel a 'give', release the trigger on the drill so that it stops. Remove the drill part.

– **BIG:** turn the dial to the correct age to set the depth of needle insertion. Hold the device against the skin, remove the safety catch and press down firmly to activate the spring-loaded needle. *Be careful only to remove the safety catch once the device is in the correct position on the patient's skin and your fingers are out of the way in order to avoid firing it through your own hand.*

■ **Remove the stylet or trochar and leave the catheter in place**. In all the above designs, there will be a central stylet or trochar which needs to be removed, leaving the catheter in place (just like when inserting a cannula and then removing the needle used to insert it). It needs to be unscrewed from inside the catheter regardless of which method you use to insert it. Dispose of the stylet in a sharps bin immediately.

■ **Aspirate a sample for testing**. This will confirm that you have sited the needle correctly as you should be able to aspirate bone marrow (which to the naked eye looks like venous blood). You can send off the bone marrow for some basic investigations (don't forget to label it as marrow not venous blood) including:

■ blood cultures

■ acid–base status

- haemoglobin
- glucose
- electrolytes
- renal function.

Do not try to run a bone marrow sample through a blood gas machine as you will break the machine.

■ **Attach extension set**. These are similar to the extension sets used for cannulas. Don't forget to prime it with 0.9% saline before attaching it.

■ **Flush using normal saline**. Flush the line with 5–10 mL of 0.9% saline for injection. If there is swelling around the needle site, this indicates that the saline is going into the soft tissues and the needle needs to be resited.

■ **Secure the needle**. If you have used a BIG to insert the needle then the red safety catch can be used to secure the needle by clipping it around the hub or the needle and then taping it to the skin. If you have used an EZ-IO they have specially designed dressings you can use to secure the needle. Other methods of making sure that the IO needle is not dislodged include the following.

– **Lots of adhesive tape**. Tear a strip of tape 4–5 cm long and tear it lengthways up to half way along the strip. Stick the whole part onto the skin and then wrap the two half strips around the hub of the needle and then stick to the skin. Repeat this a few times, sticking different lengths of tape around the hub in different places.

– **Sticking a gallipot over it**. Place a gallipot upside down over the top of

the needle and tape or bandage the gallipot securely to the skin.

– **Use syringe barrels as bolsters**. Place syringes flat against the skin along either side of the needle to act as bolsters and tape them to the skin.

– **Assign someone to hold it in place**. If you have enough people available, you can assign someone to be responsible for making sure that the IO needle is not dislodged.

■ **Administer drugs and/or fluids**. Any fluid or drug which can be given IV can also be given IO, including resuscitation drugs such as adrenaline.

■ **Remove it as soon as possible**. Given the risk of infection, IO access should be removed as soon as you manage to get adequate IV access. The maximum time an IO needle can remain *in situ* before it needs to be removed is 24 h.

 Top Tip

If you send a bone marrow sample off to the laboratory, remember to tell the laboratory that it is bone marrow not venous blood (they look very similar to the naked eye). This is so that they don't break expensive machinery which is not able to process bone marrow and also so that the haematologists are not alarmed by the presence of blast cells (which are immature cells that would indicate a leukaemia if seen in a venous blood sample but are a normal finding in bone marrow).

Nasogastric tube

For a checklist of equipment needed for insertion of a nasogastric tube see Box 6.4.

Most of the time it will be the nurses who are responsible for inserting nasogastric tubes but there may be occasions when you need to know how to do it for yourself. It is useful to be proactive in learning how to do this in a planned and calm way with supervision available rather than having to do one for the first time in the middle of the night when everyone else is busy. Ask for supervision from one of the experienced nursing staff whilst you are learning.

■ **Choose the correct type of tube.** Which tube to use depends on what you are using it for and how long the tube is going to be left *in situ*. If a nasogastric tube is being used for draining the stomach contents (e.g. in cases of bowel obstruction) then a wide tube called a Ryles tube is inserted. For feeding, you can use a tube made of pol-

yurethane if it is to be used long term (more than 10 days) or a tube made of polyvinyl chloride for short-term use (7–10 days). The range of sizes used for children is usually between 6 Fr and 10 Fr.

■ **Position the child appropriately.** For an older child, this can be done with them sitting upright. It may help to have a chair with a headrest so that they can't instinctively move their head backwards as you try to insert the tube. Younger children may be best sitting on a parent's lap with one of the parent's arms over the child's arms and one over their forehead (the same as you would do for looking in a child's throat). Babies may be best being swaddled in a blanket to hold their limbs still.

■ **Prepare the child and parents.** If possible, the child should not have anything to eat or drink for 2 h prior to insertion of a nasogastric tube (to reduce the risk of aspiration if attempted insertion causes the child to vomit). Explain to them and their parents what will happen and why the nasogastric tube is needed.

Box 6.4 Checklist of equipment needed for insertion of a nasogastric tube

■ Nasogastric tube (correct size and type)

■ pH indicator paper

■ Tape

■ Enteral syringe to aspirate stomach contents from the tube

■ Bowl of sterile water

■ A glass of water with a straw

■ Gloves

■ **Measure the length**. Each tube should be marked with measurements along the outside. Measure the distance from earlobe to tip of the nose to the xiphisternum to establish how far you should expect to insert the tube and either mark the tube with a pen or write down the length.

■ **Lubricate the tube**. Dip the whole tube in sterile warm water in order to lubricate it. Do *not* use jelly to lubricate the end as this can affect the pH reading and can also sometimes block the tube.

■ **Insert directly backwards *not upwards***. Slide the tube in *along the floor of the nasopharynx* (see Fig. 6.3). This means inserting directly backwards from the nostril towards the back of the child's head and slightly down. If you meet with a lot of resistance then do not force it; remove the tube and try the other nostril.

■ **Ask the child to swallow**. In an older child, you can give them water to

sip and ask them to swallow to help the tube down into the oesophagus. In a younger child you can give them their dummy to suck on.

■ **Make sure you are not in the lungs**. *If the child starts coughing a lot or appears in respiratory distress remove the tube immediately and completely as if this happens you are likely to be in the trachea.*

■ **Make sure you are definitely in the stomach before putting *anything down the tube***. There have been multiple National Patient Safety alerts regarding incorrectly sited nasogastric tubes because if liquid is flushed through the tube when it is in the wrong place, the patient can die as a result (for example, from feeding into the lungs). The recommended first line for confirming correct placement is by measuring the pH of aspirate from the tube. Using an enteral syringe (which is usually purple), try to aspirate from the tube and test to see if the aspirate has a pH of less than 5. *Use pH paper, which allows you to read a numerical result, not litmus paper, which does not. If you cannot get an aspirate or it is not less than 5 then do not give anything down the tube.*

■ **Remove the guidewire**. Some nasogastric tubes will have guidewires running down the inside to help with insertion. Once you have confirmed correct positioning of the tube, remove the guidewire, if there is one.

■ **Check the tube is still in the correct place**. You need to confirm that the tube is in the correct position just after you have first inserted it but

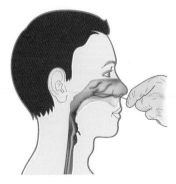

Figure 6.3 Sliding a nasogastric tube along the floor of the nasopharynx.

Box 6.5 Trouble shooting confirmation of correct nasogastric tube placement

I'm aspirating air
■ *This may mean that you are in the lungs.* Check that the child is not displaying any signs of respiratory distress and that they have normal oxygen saturation levels and respiratory rate. If there is any suggestion of respiratory distress, remove the tube immediately.

■ If the child is showing no signs of respiratory distress, you may be in the oesophagus or entrance to the stomach, not far enough in to reach the stomach contents. Try advancing the tube a few centimetres and reaspirating.

I'm not getting any aspirate
■ Try advancing the tube a few centimetres.

■ Ask the child to lie on their left side for a few minutes (in order to reposition the stomach contents) and try aspirating again.

■ If you still get nothing and the child is safe to drink, then offer them a glass of water to drink but *do not put anything down the tube* until you have confirmed its position.

■ If after this you are still not getting an aspirate, consider ordering an x-ray to confirm the correct position of the tube.

The pH of the aspirate is more than 5
■ This may mean that the tube is in the lungs or small bowel. Try withdrawing the tube by a few centimetres and taking another aspirate.

■ Check whether the child is taking medications which alter the pH of the stomach contents (e.g. proton pump inhibitors such as omeprazole or H2 receptor antagonists such as ranitidine). If this is the case you may need to order an x-ray to confirm correct positioning of the tube.

I couldn't get an aspirate and now I don't know how to interpret the x-ray
■ Incorrect interpretation of x-rays is one of the biggest problems which can lead to feeding through a tube which is in the wrong place. Some hospitals now only allow such x-rays to be acted upon once they have been reported by a radiologist to say whether or not the tube is in the correct place. You can practise interpreting them yourself with online training at www.trainingngt. co.uk. However, this uses mostly images of adult chest x-rays and you will probably need additional training to interpret neonatal films accurately. If in doubt, ask a senior colleague or radiologist for help and *do not put anything down the tube unless you are certain about its position*.

you also need to recheck before each time that you use the tube.

■ Don't forget to **involve a play specialist and praise the child afterwards**.

For a trouble-shooting guide for what to do if you can't get an aspirate with pH <5, see Box 6.5.

Lumbar puncture

For a checklist of equipment needed for lumbar puncture see Box 6.6.

This should not be something you do without supervision until you have done enough to feel competent performing the procedure without a senior colleague present. Even once you are confident performing lumbar punctures without senior supervision, you should discuss with your registrar or consultant before deciding to proceed with one. Before performing a lumbar puncture, ask yourself some important questions.

■ **Does this child have a bleeding diathesis?** Has blood been sent for a coagulation screen and are the results of this normal? Does the child have a normal platelet count? Is there any past medical or family history of bleeding disorders?

Box 6.6 Checklist of equipment needed for lumbar puncture

■ Sterile gloves

■ Sterile gown

■ Trolley

■ Antiseptic solution, e.g. 0.5% chlorhexidine

■ 1% lidocaine

■ 5 mL syringe

■ 25 G needle (usually orange) for injecting local anaesthetic

■ Sterile dressing pack (usually contains a pot for antiseptic, gauze, forceps, drape and a rubbish bag)

■ Additional sterile gauze

■ Appropriate size spinal needle

■ Manometer with tap

■ Sterile sample containers (usually universal containers – 3–4 needed, usually one for MC&S, one for protein and sometimes also one for virology, cytology or immunology)

■ Fluoride blood tube (for collecting CSF sample to be tested for glucose)

■ Dressing

■ **Does this child have raised intracranial pressure?** Any history of vomiting, reduced consciousness (including irritability, particularly in infants) or headache (particularly if worse on coughing or lying flat) should raise your suspicions. Look at the fundi for any suggestion of papilloedema and for any papillary changes. If there is any suspicion at all of the possibility of raised intracranial pressure, perform brain imaging (usually a CT scan) beforehand to rule this out before going ahead with a lumbar puncture. This is because if you perform a lumbar puncture on a child with raised intracranial pressure, it can cause herniation of posterior parts of the brain, putting pressure on the brainstem. In the early stages this can cause a ptosis and dilated pupil (due to pressure on the parasympathetic fibres around the outside of the third cranial nerve) and later can cause a respiratory arrest by compromising the respiratory centres in the brainstem. This process is sometimes known as 'coning'.

■ **Do I need to start treatment before performing a lumbar puncture?** In children who are clinically stable, it can be useful to perform a lumbar puncture prior to starting antibiotics if you suspect an infectious cause as this makes it more likely that the bacteria causing the infection can be identified on a culture of the cerebrospinal fluid (CSF). However, if the child is unwell then the priority should be to start treatment. If a child is presenting with meningism and a purpuric rash you should suspect meningococ-cal septicaemia, which is an emergency and requires immediate treatment with broad-spectrum antibiotics. *There is no time for a lumbar puncture in this circumstance and it will not change your management; start broad-spectrum antibiotics immediately.* If you are unsure whether the child is well enough then err on the side of caution and give antibiotics before performing a lumbar puncture once the child is more stable. You will still be able to get useful information from the results such as the CSF glucose, protein and white cell count, which all suggest the most likely causative organism. Performing polymerase chain reaction (PCR) tests on the sample can also be useful, particularly if you have delayed performing the lumbar puncture until the child was more stable.

Once you have answered the questions above, you can decide whether or not it is safe to proceed with a lumbar puncture. If it is, then consider the following.

■ **Prepare your equipment**. *For a checklist of equipment needed for lumbar puncture, see Box 6.6.* You will need a trolley on which to lay out all your equipment. Open the sterile dressing pack onto the trolley and unwrap the paper covering (being careful only to touch the outside part of the paper). Once you have opened this dressing pack, the paper which was wrapping it can act as a sterile field onto which you can open all your equipment. Be careful only to touch the outer wrappings and drop the items from their sterile packs onto the sterile field without touching them. Pour 0.5%

chlorhexidine solution into the sterile pot which should come in the dressing pack. Make sure that you set up a rubbish bag and sharps bin into which you can easily drop all your used equipment. The dressing packs often come with a small rubbish bag inside them which you can stick to the side of the trolley. Numbering your collection pots can help you to keep track of which pot contains the sample which was collected first (this is helpful for the laboratory to know when interpreting the results).

Top Tip

Make sure that your manometer with tap has the tap pointing in the right direction. Try turning the tap a couple of times backwards and forwards as they can sometimes be very stiff. You don't want to discover this once the manometer is attached to the patient. The tap needs to be closed at first so that the manometer fills and you can read the opening pressure. Then turn it so that the CSF drains from the bottom of the manometer a drip at a time into your sample bottles.

■ **Position the child appropriately**. Positioning the child well is crucial and can make the difference success and failure. Having an experienced nurse with you to hold the child will make an enormous difference. Lie the child on their side with their neck and hips flexed as much as possible and their back in line with the edge of the bed or couch. Most people lie the child on their left side but if you are left-handed you may find that having the child lying on their right hand side is easier for you. The child should be held behind their knees and on their shoulder, *not* their neck or head, to encourage them to flex their back as much as possible. In older children you can try performing the lumbar puncture with them sitting upright and bent forwards.

■ **Prepare the child and the parents**. For some parents it may be easier for them not to be present in the room whilst the lumbar puncture is happening. If they are, it is best to position them sitting down on the opposite side from where you and your assistant are standing (so that their child can see them and so that the parent can't see the needle going in, which they may find distressing). An age-appropriate explanation to the child about what to expect is important to help them to cope.

■ **Prepare pain relief**. Apply local anaesthetic cream on the appropriate space on the back 45–60 min before the procedure. Feel for the iliac crests and draw an imaginary line between them which should cross through the intervertebral space between L3 and L4. Feel for the spinous processes and identify the L4–L5 intervertebral space too (the next space down). *In neonates the spinal cord ends lower down so you should aim for the L4–L5 space or lower.* Put local anaesthetic cream over an area which covers both of these intervertebral spaces (if you are not successful in getting a sample initially you may have to try in both of these spaces so it makes sense to anaesthetise the skin over both). In children over 6 months you should also inject local anaesthetic just before performing the lumbar puncture. This is covered in more detail later. For older children it may be helpful to give them nitrous oxide and oxygen to breath (such as Entonox) to help with anxiety and pain.

■ **Get people to help you**. You will need at least two people to help you with performing a lumbar puncture: one to hold the child still and the other to pass you equipment.

■ **Choose the correct site**. Feel for the iliac crests and draw an imaginary line between them. In older children this should intersect the space between L3 and L4, but in smaller children (because of their smaller pelvis) this marks the L4–L5 intervertebral space and the L5–S1 intervertebral space in infants. Therefore, although in NEONATES the spinal cord ends lower down, you can still use the iliac crests as a landmark to safely guide needle insertion. Feel the spinous processes either side of the space and make sure that you can feel the gap between the two clearly. Once you have identified the correct site, it is useful to mark it. You could use a pen but this can rub off when you clean and you risk tattooing the patient if you stick the needle through the ink. A better method is to use a syringe to suck up an area of skin and leave an indent or to press the hub of a needle to make a dent in the skin.

■ **Choose the correct needle**. You should always use a spinal needle which has a stylet (a thin solid metal spike running through the inside of the needle

which is removable) because use of needles without stylets has been associated with some children developing epidermoid tumours. You will need a different length of needle depending on the size of the child but a 22 G needle is normally used. You can get smaller 25 G needles for use in NEONATES. How far you need to insert the needle in order to reach the subarachnoid space (and therefore what length of needle you will need) can be calculated using this formula:

Depth of insertion (cm)
= 0.03 × height of the child (cm)

Table 6.2 has suggestions for which size needle is likely to be suitable at which age.

■ **Take a blood glucose sample**. It is only possible to interpret the CSF glucose level if a serum sample has been taken at the same time to compare it to. This should be a laboratory sample not a finger prick bedside test. In practical terms, it is usually easiest to do this just

Table 6.2 Size of spinal needle to use for lumbar puncture according to child's age.

Age of child	Size of spinal needle
Premature infant	1 inch (23 mm) 25 G
<2 years	1.5 inch (38 mm) 22 G
2–12 years	2.5 inch (50–70 mm) 22 G
>12 years	3.5 inch (90 mm) 22 G

before you perform the lumbar puncture rather than afterwards.

■ **Prepare yourself**. Lumbar punctures should be done under sterile conditions so ensure that you wash your hands thoroughly and dress in a sterile gown and sterile gloves. Be careful only to touch other things which are sterile once you have put on your gown and gloves. This includes avoiding touching the patient's skin before you have cleaned it (you can use forceps to hold gauze for cleaning in order to manage this).

■ **Clean the skin**. If you haven't already done so, ask your assistant to pour 0.5% chlorhexidine into the sterile pot which comes in the dressing pack. Soak sterile gauze in the chlorhexidine and use it to clean over the planned puncture site and the surrounding skin, working outwards in circular motions.

■ **Inject local anaesthetic**. With your assistant helping you (by opening and holding the vial), draw up 3–5 mL of 1% lidocaine into a syringe (don't forget to check the drug name and use-by date on the vial). Warn the child that the local anaesthetic may sting and inject slowly just under the skin over your planned puncture site, drawing back on the syringe before injecting to ensure that you are not in a blood vessel. Gradually infiltrate deeper into the tissues with local anaesthetic along the track of where the spinal needle will go, drawing back on the syringe each time before injecting. You will need to allow a few minutes for the local anaesthetic to work.

■ **Insert the spinal needle**. Feel again exactly where you want to put

your needle (touching only skin which has been cleaned) and then insert the needle with the bevel upwards. The needle should be completely parallel with the surface on which the child is lying (i.e. horizonatal) and advanced so that it is pointing slightly towards the umbilicus. Advance slowly and firmly until you feel a 'give' as the needle passes into the subarachnoid space.

■ **Withdraw stylet and wait for CSF to drain**. Even when you are in the right place, CSF comes out really slowly so be patient. It also isn't easy to spot unless you're watching carefully as it should be colourless. Once you have removed the stylet, make yourself count to 10 slowly before deciding that the CSF is not coming out and readjusting.

■ **No CSF?** Put the stylet back inside the needle and advance a tiny bit before removing the stylet again to check and wait for CSF. If you still get nothing coming out, try rotating the needle slightly without moving it further in or out as this can sometimes align the bevel of the needle with the flow of CSF and allow you to get a sample. If you're still not having any luck, try withdrawing the needle very slightly. If you feel like you are hitting bone with your needle, come out almost to the skin and then change the angle of your needle before trying to advance it again. *Make sure that the stylet is always in when you are moving the needle; only take it out to check if CSF is flowing and collect a sample.*

■ **Measure opening pressure**. In some cases this may not be needed but if you are planning to measure the opening pressure, attach your manometer to the needle once you have seen a drop of CSF. Wait until the level has stopped rising to take a reading but bear in mind that if the child is moving or crying, you will not get an accurate reading. If you have used a manometer you can drip CSF from the bottom of the manometer into the collection pots by turning the three-way tap.

■ **Collect a CSF sample!** Don't forget to collect in the right order if you have numbered the collection pots beforehand. You will usually need about 6–10 drops of CSF per sample bottle.

■ **Reinsert the stylet before withdrawing the needle**. This may help to reduce the incidence of headaches following lumbar puncture.

■ **Apply pressure over the site and apply a dressing**. Once you have

removed the needle, apply pressure over the puncture site with sterile gauze. If you have it available at your hospital, use operating site spray to seal the needle hole. Apply a sterile dressing.

■ **Postprocedure care**. Ideally the child should lie flat for the next few hours (or as long as possible!) in order to minimise the risk of a headache. They should have hourly neurological observations and blood pressure measurement for the next few hours too.

Urinary catheter insertion

For a list of equipment needed for insertion of a urinary catheter see Box 6.7.

Urinary catheters are sometimes done as an 'in-out' catheter to collect a

---

Box 6.7 Checklist of equipment needed for insertion of a urinary catheter

■ Trolley

■ Apron

■ Sterile gloves

■ Catheter pack (usually contains sterile gauze, a gallipot, kidney dish, forceps and a rubbish bag)

■ Antiseptic solution (e.g. 0.9% saline or 0.5% chlorhexidine)

■ Anaesthetic lubricating gel (e.g. 0.1% lidocaine gel)

■ Urinary catheter (choose the correct size and male or female)

■ Urine collection bag

■ Sterile water or 0.9% saline for balloon inflation

■ 5 or 10 mL syringe

■ Sterile urine specimen container

■ Tape

---

urine sample (i.e. the catheter is put in, sample taken and then removed immediately). They are also used in critically ill children in order to accurately assess fluid balance by measuring the urine output.

■ **Choose the right size of catheter**. The urethra is much shorter in females than in males and therefore different catheters are used depending on the sex of your patient, so make sure that you've checked and have the right type. Then you need to decide on a size (which refers to the diameter of the catheter). The French gauge system is used for catheter sizes which is commonly abbreviated to either Fr or Ch (both are the same measurement). A 6 Fr or 8 Fr catheter is usually appropriate for babies, 8 Fr or 10 Fr for most school-age children and 10 Fr or 12 Fr for older children. This is a rough estimate and it may be a good idea to take a couple of different sizes with you to the bedside to assess which looks to be the most appropriate size to use.

■ **Prepare your equipment**. Open your catheter pack on top of the trolley (touching only the outside of the sterile wrapping) to create a sterile field and then open all your equipment onto it. Take care only to touch the outside of the packaging and let the equipment fall onto the sterile field without touching it. Pour some sterile 0.9% saline into the pot in the dressing pack so that it is ready to use. Stick the rubbish bag to the side of the trolley so that it is easy to access.

■ **Prepare the child and the parents**. If the child is old enough and well enough to understand, explain to them in simple terms what will happen and why

the catheter is needed (including how long the catheter is likely to stay in for).

■ **Position the child appropriately**. The easiest position is for the child to be lying supine. For girls, they will need to have their legs bent and hips flexed. You will need an assistant to hold the child still.

■ **Involve a play specialist**. If the child is old enough and alert enough to understand what is happening, involve a play specialist to distract them during the procedure.

■ **Prepare yourself**. Once you have set up your equipment, wash your hands thoroughly and put on an apron and sterile gloves. Throughout the whole procedure, you should try to keep one hand (usually your dominant hand) 'clean'. This means that you do not touch the child's skin with that hand so that the glove remains sterile for handling the urinary catheter. If this is too tricky or you forget, you can always

 Top Tip

Don't forget to have a sterile kidney dish or pot ready to catch the urine which will pour out once the catheter reaches the bladder. Also, babies and young children may urinate whilst you are cleaning so be ready to catch it with a sterile pot if this happens (as if the catheter was only being done in order to collect a sample then it will no longer be necessary if you can get a clean catch sample).

change to a new pair of sterile gloves just before inserting the catheter.

■ **Clean around the urethra**. You can use sterile gauze soaked in 0.9% saline for cleaning and the forceps provided in the dressing pack to hold the gauze.

– For boys, gently retract the foreskin with one hand (but don't force it, especially in infants). Clean around the urethral opening, moving outwards to clean the whole of the glans of the penis.

– For girls, separate the labia with one hand. Clean around the urethral opening and the labial folds using one downwards wiping motion from the urethra towards the anus with each swab before discarding and using a fresh one.

■ **Prepare pain relief**. You can use anaesthetic gel (such as Instillagel) to numb and lubricate the urethra. Instil 1–5 mL into the urethra and then wait for 5 min for the anaesthetic to work.

■ **Check the catheter balloon works**. While you're waiting for the anaesthetic gel to work, you can check that the balloon on the catheter is working by inflating and then deflating it again. Most paediatric catheters require 5 mL of saline or sterile water to inflate the balloon, whereas adult-sized catheters usually require 10 mL. Check on the catheter pack or the catheter itself as it will tell you the volume required.

■ **Place sterile drape over the child**. Some of the drapes provided in catheter packs now come with a hole already in the centre but others do not. If there is no hole in the drape, tear off the folded corner to create one and then place the drape over the child.

■ **Insert the catheter**.

– For boys, hold the penis upright so that it is pointing towards the ceiling as this helps to straighten out the urethra and make the catheter easier to advance. Continue to advance the catheter slowly until you meet resistance (which should mean that you have reached the bladder neck) and make sure that you have the other end of the catheter in a kidney dish. When this happens, rotate the catheter gently backwards and forwards until the sphincter relaxes and you can advance the catheter through into the bladder. If this doesn't work, you can try lowering the penis 90° (so that it is pointing towards the child's feet) or ask the child to cough or try to pass urine. *Do not force it if you are meeting a lot of resistance*. If you still can't pass the catheter, try getting someone experienced to help you.

– For girls, part the labia with one hand and gently insert the catheter into the urethral opening with the other. Slowly advance the catheter, making sure that the other end is in a sterile kidney dish (to catch the urine). You may need to angle slightly upwards as if towards the umbilicus in order to advance the catheter.

■ **Inflate the balloon**. Once there is urine flowing, you know that you have reached the bladder so hold the catheter in place (being careful not to accidentally withdraw it slightly) and inflate the balloon. If this causes the child pain then it is likely that you are in the urethra and you must deflate the balloon immediately, try advancing the catheter slightly further and then try again. Once you have fully inflated the balloon, gently pull back on the catheter until you feel resistance (so that you know that the balloon is resting against the bladder sphincter).

■ **Attach a urine collection bag**. If the catheter has been inserted for accurate fluid balance monitoring you may wish to attach a bag which allows for measurement of an hourly urine output.

■ **Tape the catheter down**. Taping the catheter to the inside of the child's thigh can help to stop it from being accidentally pulled. Make sure to leave enough slack to allow for movement of the child's leg without the catheter tugging.

■ **Measure and document the volume of urine drained**. This is important to note down if the catheter is being inserted for accurate fluid balance management or because of urinary retention.

■ **Remove the catheter as soon as possible**. The presence of an indwelling urinary catheter makes the child more vulnerable to contracting a urinary tract infection. Reassess the need for the catheter daily and remove it as soon as possible.

Suprapubic urine sample

For a list of equipment needed for taking a suprapubic urine sample see Box 6.8.

Suprapubic aspiration is a method which can be used to collect urine samples from babies and young toddlers (usually only done in children under 2 years). It remains the gold standard for obtaining a urine specimen for children in whom the result is very important as it has a very low risk of sample contamination, but it should only be used if non-invasive methods have been unsuccessful.

■ **Have a urine pot to hand**. Before you even undo the nappy, make sure that

---

Box 6.8   Checklist of equipment needed for taking a suprapubic urine sample

■ Sterile gloves

■ Alcohol skin wipes

■ 10 mL syringe

■ 23 G needle (usually blue)

■ Sterile urine specimen pot

■ Cotton wool

■ A plaster for sticking over the puncture after the procedure you have a sterile urine specimen pot to hand as even this can prompt a baby to urinate. You may be able to collect a clean catch sample, meaning that you no longer need to do a suprapubic aspirate.

■ **Prepare the parents**. Explain the procedure, what will happen and why it is necessary. Warn parents that their child may pass a small amount of blood in the urine following the procedure.

■ **Position the child appropriately**. It is best to have the child lying supine with an assistant helping to hold the child's hips abducted (this will also make it easier to catch a urine sample if the child urinates).

■ **Use a bladder scanner to check if there is enough urine**. It is recommended in the NICE guidelines on urinary tract infection that an ultrasound scan of the bladder should be performed before collecting a suprapubic aspirate to check that there is a sufficient volume of urine in the bladder (National Collaborating Centre for Women's and Children's Health 2007). This should increase your chances of success on first attempt. If there is more than 20 mL of urine present in the bladder then you are likely to be successful. If not, then wait and try scanning again a little later (remembering to leave the parents with a sterile pot in case the child passes urine in the meantime). Different bladder scanners vary in how they work so if you are unsure how to use the one at your hospital, ask for help. Generally, the following usually applies.

– **Select the correct setting**. Many will have different settings for male or female or different ones for adults and children. Select the correct settings for your patient.

– **Apply ultrasound jelly suprapubically**. This feels cold and may prompt the baby to start passing urine – be ready to catch it!

– **Hold the probe at 90° to the skin suprapubically**.

■ **Percuss to identify the bladder**. There should be dullness to percussion suprapubically when the bladder is full.

■ **Put on sterile gloves and an apron**.

■ **Clean the skin**. Using an alcohol wipe, clean the skin over the anterior abdominal wall in the suprapubic region.

■ **Insert the needle**. Aim in the midline (imagine a straight line between the umbilicus and the pubic symphysis) roughly 1 cm above the pubic bone (in the lower abdominal skin crease). The needle should be inserted at 90° to the abdominal wall (which usually means that the needle is not completely vertical but instead angled slightly so that the end of the syringe is angled slightly towards the feet). Advance slowly, aspirating as you advance and stopping as soon as urine starts to fill the syringe. You may need to advance almost to the hub of the needle. If you don't manage to aspirate any urine, withdraw the needle almost to the skin and then try advancing at a slightly different angle.

■ **Press over the puncture site**. Remove the needle and then press over the puncture site with a piece of cotton wool before applying a plaster over the site.

■ **Transfer the urine to a sterile sample pot**. Make sure that you do not contaminate the specimen in the process. Transfer the specimen immediately from the syringe into a urine specimen pot.

■ **Not getting any urine?** If you have not managed to aspirate any urine, you can try hydrating the child and returning later or performing an in-out catheter instead.

Mantoux test

For a list of equipment needed for performing a Mantoux test see Box 6.9.

This test is still used for some patients in the diagnosis of suspected *Mycobacterium tuberculosis* infection. The principle is that a small amount of a protein from the mycobacterium is injected into the skin and if that individual has previously been exposed to *M. tuberculosis* then they will develop induration (thickening) of the skin at the site of the injection. This method of testing is less useful in people who have been vaccinated with BCG or who are infected with another form of Mycobacterium as there is a certain amount of cross-reactive action of the immune system against these. It can

also produce false-negative results in children whose immune reaction is poor (for example, as a result of immunosuppression). However, it is still often used to aid diagnosis in children presenting with symptoms suggestive of *M. tuberculosis* infection and to screen children who are at high risk or to whom you plan to give the BCG vaccine so it is important to know how to administer the tuberculin and 'read' the Mantoux results.

> **Top Tip**
>
> This is a notifiable disease so if you do suspect tuberculosis clinically, don't forget to contact your local public health agency immediately. Do not wait for the result of the Mantoux or any other tests before you call them. They want to know as early as possible so that they can take protective action to prevent potential spread of the disease.

Injecting tuberculin

■ **Prepare the child and the parents**. Explain what the procedure involves and that they will need to return in 48–72 h for the result of the test to

---

Box 6.9   Checklist of equipment needed for performing a Mantoux test

■ Gloves

■ 1 mL syringe

■ 25 G or 26 G short bevelled needle (such as those used for insulin injection)

■ Tuberculin purified protein derivative (needs to be kept in the fridge)

be interpreted. Warn the child that it will sting as the injection is given and that they may have some mild itching or swelling of the site afterwards but to avoid scratching it if possible.

■ **Wash only if necessary**. If the skin is visibly dirty then ask the child to wash their arm with soap and water but otherwise there is no need to clean the skin before injection.

■ **Draw up 0.1 mL of tuberculin purified protein derivative**. This comes in different strengths. Tuberculin purified protein derivative (PPD) is measured in tuberculin units (TU). The standard strength which should be used for Mantoux testing is 2 TU/0.1 mL and comes in a little glass vial. Check the vial to make sure that the tuberculin PPD is within the use-by date and is the correct strength. Then draw up 0.1 mL into a syringe and expel any air bubbles. Previously, a different dose of tuberculin was used for children who had been vaccinated with BCG, but 2 TU is now routinely used in all patients. Occasionally, a 10 TU dose is given if a second Mantoux test is needed for clinical diagnosis (Salisbury et al. 2006).

■ **Choose the correct site**. The normal site to use for the Mantoux test is the flexor surface of the left forearm, about a third of the way along from the elbow to the hand (see Fig. 6.4).

■ **Inject the tuberculin intradermally**. Stretch the skin taut between your thumb and first finger and then insert the needle at a very shallow angle (almost parallel with the surface of the skin), with the bevel of the needle facing

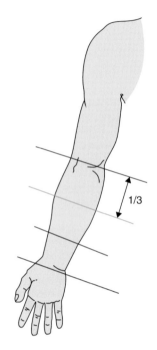

Figure 6.4 Mantoux test. The orange line indicates the correct area to use as the site for the test.

upwards. You only need to advance the needle 3–4 mm (just so that the entire bevel of the needle is fully under the skin) and the needle tip should be visible through the skin. Release the stretched skin and then slowly inject the tuberculin. If the needle is in the right place you should feel quite a lot of resistance as you inject and a small, firm bleb of liquid should form in the skin.

■ **Make an appointment to check the results**. Arrange an appointment with the child and their parents in the next 48–72 h in order to look at the child's arm and assess the reaction to the injection.

'Reading' the Mantoux test results

■ **Check the injection timing**. Ideally you should be assessing the outcome 48–72 h after the tuberculin injection was given although it is sometimes possible to gain a valid reading up to 96 h after the injection.

■ **Measure the raised area**. What you need to measure and record in the notes is the diameter of the 'indurated' area of skin. This means the area of skin which is raised and you can feel when you run your finger over the forearm. Any surrounding area of redness is irrelevant and should not be included in your measurement. Feel around with your finger and mark dots at the edges of the raised area. If the area is an irregular shape then take the widest measurement and record the numerical value in the notes along with how many hours after the tuberculin injection you are reading the result.

■ **Interpret the result**. The size of the indurated area dictates whether the Mantoux test is deemed to be negative or positive. There is a grey area in terms of where the cut-off should be and therefore it is vital to always clearly record in the notes the numerical value for your reading, not just 'positive' or 'negative'. If the indurated area is less than 6 mm diameter then this is a negative result and more than 15 mm is a strongly

positive result and suggests tuberculosis infection. An indurated area of between 6 mm and 15 mm is positive but can suggest a number of different causes such as previous BCG vaccination, previous TB infection or exposure to non-tuberculous mycobacteria. Therefore, for these results it is important to seek advice from senior colleagues about management based on the clinical picture. *There are false positives and negatives for this test so it is important to interpret it in the context of the clinical history.*

Peak flow

Peak flow testing can only really be done reliably by children who are 6 or 7 years or older. Peak flow measurement forms part of the classification of acute asthma attacks into moderate, severe or life-threatening although in reality, if the child is acutely unwell treatment is started without measuring the peak flow. *For more about the management of acute asthma see Chapter 5 – Common Paediatric Emergencies.* Peak flow measurement is also important for long-term management of children with asthma to ensure that their treatment is optimal.

■ **Attach a clean mouthpiece**. Use disposable mouthpieces with built-in filters and attach a clean one to the peak flow device.

■ **Ask the child to stand**. This will make sure that they can breathe in as fully as possible to get an accurate reading.

■ **Check the pointer**. Make sure that the red pointer is set to zero and that the child's fingers will not be in the way as it moves.

■ **Good seal around the mouth-piece**. Check that the child has a good seal around the mouthpiece and that their tongue is not blocking the mouthpiece.

■ **Short, sharp breath out**. Ask the child to take as big a breath in as they can and then to breathe out as quickly and forcefully as they can in one short, sharp breath. With younger children, you can ask them to pretend that they are the big bad wolf trying to blow down the house built of bricks so they can eat the little piggies.

■ **Demonstrate yourself first**. It can then be helpful to demonstrate yourself, without the actual device or with a different mouthpiece, so that the child knows what you want them to do.

■ **Take three readings**. Get the child to do three different peak flow measurements and record the *highest* of the three results as the child's peak flow result.

■ **Discount attempts with poor technique**. If the child coughs or spits into the peak flow meter this can give falsely high results so if this happens then discount that reading.

■ **Plot the result**. Plotting the result on a peak flow chart can give useful information about whether or not the child is improving. Remember to also record the reading in the notes. If you are measuring a peak flow in clinic, when the child is well, consider recording it as the child's personal best if it is higher than previously recorded results and the child has grown significantly since their previous personal best was recorded.

Hand-held spirometry

Many units will now have hand-held electronic spirometers so that you can perform lung function tests at the bedside. Don't forget to take something to write down the results on if the machine doesn't automatically store or print readings.

Explaining to the child what they need to do and encouraging them to use maximal effort is the most difficult part of the process. The technique is similar to that for peak flow but after doing the short, sharp breath out (as for peak flow), the child needs to continue breathing out for as long as they can until their lungs are completely empty. Some devices will have an animation which can be used as visual encouragement. This is sometimes referred to as 'computerised incentive spirometry'. Examples of such animations include a child blowing up a piece of bubble gum or a balloon blowing across the screen or an animation which looks like an accelerator dial for older children (if there are several different ones available, offer the child the choice of which one they would like to use). These visual cues help to ensure that the child keeps breathing out for as long as possible and puts in maximal effort in order to get accurate vital capacity and forced expiratory volume measurements. If you do not have a device with a visual aid, you can ask the child to imagine that they are trying to blow out all the candles on an enormous birthday cake. Using their parents to encourage them as well and trying to turn it into a fun game can help.

Children under 6 can rarely perform spirometry reliably and even older children may need several practice attempts before you get a reliable result.

Setting up a nebuliser

There may be times when it is useful to know how to set up a nebuliser (such as for a child who is acutely unwell in the emergency department at a time when all the nurses are looking after other sick children).

Nebulisers can be driven by air or by oxygen. Usually, if the child is requiring a nebuliser (such as nebulised adrenaline or salbutamol), they are likely to also have an oxygen requirement so it is probably good practice to drive all nebulisers with oxygen unless you have a good reason not to.

The principle of nebulised therapy is creating a vapour of medication which is inhaled by the patient. The liquid medication is poured into a container attached to the bottom of the facemask. Oxygen (or in some cases air) is then pushed through the liquid, forming a mist which the patient then breathes in from the mask.

You need to set the oxygen flow rate at between 6 and 10 litres per minute to provide enough power for the medication to form a vapour.

Inhaler technique and using a spacer

The most effective method of delivering inhaled medications is using a metered dose inhaler (MDI) and a spacer device. This is much more effective at delivering medication to the airways than an inhaler alone or a nebuliser.

Here are some things to consider when advising on the use of an inhaler with a spacer.

■ **How old is the child?** The most effective way of delivering medication to the lungs is to use a spacer with a mouthpiece but younger children will not be able to do this effectively. For children under the age of 3, it is more effective to use a spacer with a mask which should be fitted firmly over their nose and mouth to form a seal.

■ **What will they actually use?** The large volumatic spacers are the most effective at delivering medication to the airways and can be useful when children are taking inhalers at home. However, they are bulky and difficult to carry around so an aerochamber or optichamber (which are much smaller) can be easier for taking to school or going away from home.

■ **Shake the inhaler.** The MDI needs to be shaken each time before it is pressed in order to ensure that it delivers the full dose of the medication.

■ **Put the inhaler in the end of the spacer**.

■ **Get the child ready.** Either ask the child to form a tight seal around the mouthpiece with their lips or place the facemask over the child's nose and mouth so that it forms a seal with the face.

■ **Press the inhaler to release a dose of medication into the spacer**.

■ **Ask the child to breathe in and out as normal**. There is no need to take deep breaths in as the speed of this can deposit a lot of the medication at the back of the throat instead of getting to the airways. The child just needs to take 5–10 normal, relaxed breaths in and out. If the spacer starts to make a squeaky noise this means that they are breathing in and out too vigorously.

 Top Tip

If a child needs four puffs of an inhaler, people often make the mistake of pressing the device four times in a row and thinking that they have delivered enough medication. Each puff of medication must be delivered one at a time via the spacer and the inhaler needs to be shaken between each dose.

■ **Try to make it less of a battle**. With young children, parents can find it really difficult to deliver inhaled medications as they struggle to get the child to co-operate. This can mean that they avoid giving the medication at all or that they give it whilst the child is crying, which makes delivery to the airways much less effective. Decorating the spacer with colourful stickers and incorporating giving inhalers into a routine (such as sitting

down to read a story) or turning it into a game may all be helpful in getting the child to co-operate.

Intramuscular injections (for immunisations)

Although this is unlikely to form part of your routine day-to-day practice, it is important to know how to do this in case you need to give intramuscular (IM) adrenaline in an emergency for anaphylaxis or if you are asked to give a child an immunisation (which is often done by the doctors rather than the nurses on the ward, for some reason).

 Top Tip

Intramuscular injections are contraindicated in children with coagulation disorders. Make sure that you check the patient's past medical history, latest blood coagulation results and platelet counts before giving an IM injection.

■ **Choose the correct site**. For babies, the best site to inject is the lateral aspect of the midthigh. For older children, you can inject into the deltoid muscle (outer aspect of upper arm). The upper outer quadrant of the buttocks is sometimes also used but there is concern that this can potentially cause damage to the sciatic nerve.

■ **Choose the correct size needle**. Use a 23 G, 1 inch needle (usually has a blue hub). This size will be OK for most children as you can vary the depth of insertion depending on their size. Bear in mind that if you bunch the muscle before injecting, you will need to inject slightly deeper to reach the muscle. You may need a longer needle for obese children with a lot of subcutaneous fat.

■ **Clean the skin with an alcohol wipe**.

■ **Bunch the bulk of the muscle between your thumb and first finger**.

■ **Insert the needle at 90° to the skin and deep into the muscle**. Do this as quickly and smoothly as possible in order to minimise pain. Because there are no major blood vessels at the recommended sites, there is no need to aspirate before injecting.

How to use an Epipen/Anapen

For information about the emergency management of anaphylaxis see Chapter 5 – Common Paediatric Emergencies.

For a demonstration on how to use an Epipen, see Video 2.

You need to know how to use these properly for children presenting with anaphylaxis; you may also come across cases in the community when this is essential to know.

Many hospitals keep preloaded adrenaline syringes of some kind for giving intramuscularly in emergencies. *Find out which ones are used at your trust and where they are kept; you don't want to be finding out this information for the first time in an emergency.*

■ **Take off the safety caps**. Epipens only have a safety cap at one end, Anapens have safety caps over both ends of the device.

■ **Hold the child's leg still**.

■ **Jab the needle end of the pen firmly into the mid, outer thigh**. In Epipen devices the act of pressing the device against the thigh activates the needle. In Anapens you need to press the red button at the end of the device.

■ **Make sure that you hear a click**. If there is no click, then you haven't pressed hard enough to activate the needle so you need to press more firmly against the thigh.

■ **Hold the pen in place for 10 sec**. Do not move it for 10 sec in order to allow sufficient time for all the adrenaline to be injected.

Changing a nappy

When you are working on the postnatal ward doing baby checks, you will probably find that you are changing quite a lot of nappies. With parents who are willing and able to, you can step aside and let them finish off changing the nappy after a baby check but particularly for women who have had caesarean sections and are finding it difficult to move, it is often much appreciated by the parents if you change it for them. It sounds like a pretty straightforward task but can feel really clumsy to do at first, particularly with the parents watching you. Here are some tips to help you look like you know what you're doing.

■ **Hold the baby's feet in one hand**. Babies wriggle their legs a lot and so unless you hold their feet whilst you're changing their nappy, they can end up getting their heels covered in poo and then spreading it everywhere. In order to avoid this, undo the sticky bits on the nappy and then put one hand around both of their ankles before you open the nappy. Then lift their legs in the air (so that they are out of the way whilst you clean their bottom).

■ **Watch out for weeing**. Often, when you take off the nappy babies decide that it is a great time to pass urine. Make sure that you have a clean nappy quickly to hand to avoid being sprayed.

■ **Sticky, sticky meconium**. Babies will still be passing meconium (rather than normal baby poo) at the stage you are doing their newborn baby check. This stuff is like tar and can be really tricky to clean off. One trick which can work quite well is using the clean part of the nappy to wipe off as much as possible first. Baby wipes are really good for getting meconium off but if these aren't available then cotton wool soaked in warm water can work too. Remember to only ever wipe from front to back in girls to minimise the risk of urinary tract infection.

■ **Avoid the umbilical cord**. When putting on a clean nappy, fasten it so that the umbilical cord is outside the nappy so that it does not get covered in urine. This may mean that you have to fold down the top of the nappy a little bit.

References

National Collaborating Centre for Women's and Children's Health (2007) *Urinary Tract Infection in Children: Diagnosis, Treatment and Long-Term Management*. Royal College of Obstetricians and Gynaecologists, London.

Salisbury D, Ramsay M, Noakes K (2006) *Immunisation against Infectious Disease*. Stationery Office, Norwich.

Shah P, Herbozo C, Aliwalas L, Shah V (2012) Breastfeeding or breast milk for procedural pain in infants. *Cochrane Database Syst Rev* **12**: CD004950.

Chapter 7
PRESCRIBING IN CHILDREN

General principles

Prescribing for children can be quite daunting at first as it differs significantly from adult medicine and the doses used may not be as familiar to you. The golden rule when prescribing for children is to ask for help if in any doubt. The children's ward should have a dedicated pharmacist who is a specialist for children; get to know them well – they are extremely helpful. Prescribing errors are common and can be very dangerous; see Box 7.1 for key safety points to remember when prescribing for children.

Some key things to remember when prescribing for children.

■ **There is a separate British National Formulary (BNF) for prescribing in children (BNFc).** It is an indispensible resource and amongst other useful material, at the very back of the book it contains tables for estimating body surface area using a child's weight and a guide table for ideal weight.

■ **Doses differ depending on the child's age and weight** and some drugs doses are calculated using body surface area (see BNFc for body surface area table).

■ **The maximum dose which can be given is the adult dose.** So if the calculation of milligrams per kilogram comes to a total of 420 mg but the adult dose is 400 mg, you would prescribe 400 mg for the child.

■ **Use ideal body weight for overweight children.** If a child is obese, the dose must be calculated based on their ideal body weight to ensure that it is appropriate for their organ function at that age. Check the guide table in the BNFc or growth charts to estimate ideal body weight.

■ **Round up or down to a sensible amount.** Bear in mind when prescribing how the dose will be measured by the person drawing up and administering the medications; it may be more sensible to round up or down from the calculated dose. For example, co-amoxiclav comes in vials of 600 mg so if your calculation comes to 595 mg then rounding up and prescribing 600 mg is much more sensible. For unit sizes, check the BNFc, ask the pharmacist or the ward sister.

■ **Don't forget to specify the strength if prescribing by volume.** Some drugs in the BNFc are given as volumes (mL) rather than doses (mg)

The Hands-on Guide to Practical Paediatrics, First Edition. Rebecca Hewitson and Caroline Fertleman.
© 2014 John Wiley & Sons, Ltd. Published 2014 by John Wiley & Sons, Ltd.
Companion Website: www.wileyhandsonguides.com/paediatrics

Box 7.1 Don't forget when prescribing

- Never prescribe whilst distracted
- Allergies
- Calculate dose by weight or body surface area
- Minimum number of doses per day
- Some drugs are quoted as *mg/kg/dose* and some *mg/kg/day*
- Never exceed adult dose
- Write 'micrograms' and 'units' in full (don't abbreviate and risk drug errors)
- Always check the BNFc
- Double check with pharmacist or senior colleague/paediatrician if unsure
- Use ideal body weight to calculate doses for obese children
- Be careful and clear in your use of decimal points
- Be conscious of the potential for ten-fold prescribing errors (some of your patients may weigh 5 kg whilst others weigh 50 kg

and parents also tend to describe their child's medication in volume (mL or spoonfuls), but you need to find out the strength of the preparation before you prescribe as some medicines come in different strengths, e.g. furosemide solution is available in four strengths from 5 mg/5 mL up to 50 mg/5 mL. This is particularly important when the preparation has been specifically tailored for the patient.

■ Many drugs are prescribed 'off-licence'. Most drugs have come to market following testing on adults but their use has never been researched in children. This means that many, even very commonly used drugs are prescribed 'off-licence' when they are prescribed for children. This does not make much difference in practical terms and the BNFc will list those which are not formally licensed for use in children

(and then list a whole load of doses for that drug in different age groups!). It is useful to be aware of this so that you can consider trying to use a drug which is licensed for children in situations where there are several possible alternatives to choose from. The Medicines for Children Research Network has been created in order to co-ordinate and increase the volume of

 Top Tip

The usual routine when dispensing medications is for two nurses to check the prescription before administering any drug. Therefore, if a nurse questions one of your prescriptions, listen to what they have to say and recheck it very carefully yourself or with one of your colleagues.

much-needed research into medicines for children. Its webpage (www.mcrn.org.uk) has some useful pages for parents and children about what research trials involve and how they can help improve care for children by taking part.

Getting children to actually take what you prescribe

A particularly important consideration in paediatric prescribing is compliance. It's all very well writing a medication on the drug chart but if the child spits it all out, the drug won't be doing much other than making a mess!

Some suggestions to aid compliance with medication include the following.

■ **Try to keep regimes to a maximum of twice daily where possible.**

■ **Use the formulation that is the best tolerated -** ask your ward pharmacist and nursing staff which formulations are best tolerated and if a particular drug can be disguised in something more tasty. In some instances, drugs are so poorly tolerated due to their taste that they are avoided completely in some paediatric departments (e.g. flucloxacillin).

■ **Explain what the medication is for.** In older children, explaining to them in simple terms what their medications are for can aid compliance. Always involve parents in decisions about medications in younger children. Teenagers

may prefer not to have their parents involved and it is important to respect their requests where possible. *See Chapter 3 on assessment of Gillick Competence and consent in teenagers.*

■ **Help children and families to understand more about their medications.** The Medicines for Children website (www.medicinesforchildren.org.uk) is a fantastic resource. It contains lots of information about specific medications and more general principles of giving medication to children. You can print information leaflets about specific drugs for parents or refer them directly to the website itself.

■ **Think about discharge plans.** Consider how medications are going to be taken once the child has gone home. For outpatient or discharge medication, consider the timing of doses (avoid school-time doses if at all possible) and also prescribe doses rounded to easily measurable quantities (e.g. 5 mL spoonfuls) where possible.

Fluids

For initial intravenous (IV) fluid resuscitation of children in shock or with diabetic ketoacidosis, please also see Chapter 5 – Common Paediatric Emergencies.

Children who need to be kept nil by mouth or who are severely dehydrated will need IV fluids. When prescribing maintenance fluids (e.g. whilst a child is awaiting surgery), you need to meet their baseline requirements of fluids, electrolytes and glucose. For children who are dehydrated, assess the clinical severity of dehydration and from this, how much fluid they will need to be given in addition to their baseline requirements. Parenteral (i.e. oral or nasogastric) fluid is a much safer option where possible so only prescribe fluid intravenously when absolutely necessary.

Maintenance fluids

Please note that the fluid regimes below do not apply to babies who are less than 1 year old. For maintenance fluid regimes in babies under 1 year see Chapter 9 – Neonates.

For maintenance fluids in children, many hospitals use 0.9% sodium chloride and 5% dextrose, i.e. the bag contains equal parts 0.9% saline and 5% dextrose. 5% dextrose with 'half normal saline' (i.e. 0.45% saline and 5% dextrose) is rarely used now as it can cause hyponatraemia. Fluids are normally only available in 500 mL bags on the children's ward. Add 10 mmol of potassium to each 500 mL of fluid to meet the daily requirements for children who have normal potassium levels. This is a commonly used regime but check your local hospital guidelines for the preferred fluid maintenance regime.

> ### Top Tip
>
> As for other medications, IV fluids should not exceed the adult dose, regardless of the child's weight. Maximum volume of *maintenance* fluids for children is 2000 mL for girls and 2500 mL for boys.

See Box 7.2 for worked examples of calculations for maintenance fluid.

Replacement therapy

Oral replacement of fluids is the safest option where possible for a child with mild-to-moderate dehydration. If a child is not tolerating fluids orally you should also consider giving fluid via nasogastric (NG) tube before thinking of IV fluid replacement.

For trials of oral replacement, use oral rehydration salts solution (a common brand is Dioralyte). Aim to correct the child's fluid deficit over a period of 4 h; this can either be given as a small volume every 10 min or as a continuous NG infusion (see example 1 in Box 7.4 for calculations).

For children who require IV fluids, you need to consider how dehydrated they are and how quickly to replace their fluid deficit.

Traditionally, a child's additional fluid requirements are calculated by assessing their percentage dehydration. This is what people mean when they mention that a child needs 'MAINTENANCE PLUS 5%'. If you are saying you think that a child is 5% dehydrated, this means that you think they have lost 5% of their body weight as a result of fluid loss. *Every 1 g of body weight lost is the equivalent of 1 mL of fluid loss.* This means that if you have a recent weight for the child when they were well and today's weight, you can calculate how much weight (and therefore how much fluid) they have lost. You then know exactly how much fluid they will need *in addition* to the normal maintenance requirements (as mentioned above). This is much more commonly used for babies, who are weighed frequently, but can be used for children if, for example, they have recently been weighed at an outpatient appointment.

 Top Tip

Remembering that 1 g body weight is equivalent to 1 ml of fluid is key to understanding replacement fluids. It means that you don't need to memorise any formulas because how you calculate replacement fluid becomes obvious. *Remember to always do the calculations using the child's weight in grams to give you the volume in millilitres.* See the examples in Box 7.4 for workings.

Next, consider how quickly you plan to correct the child's fluid deficit. As a general rule, if a child is 5% dehydrated or less, you can correct the deficit over a period of 24 h and if a child is more than 5% dehydrated, you correct over a period of 48 h. Major exceptions to this are children who are significantly hypernatraemic or children with diabetic ketoacidosis (DKA) whose fluid loss should be replaced over 48 h or more (see *Chapter 5 – Common Paediatric Emergencies*).

If you do not have a recent weight for a child, you can estimate their percentage dehydration based on clinical signs (Box 7.3). The NICE guidelines on diarrhoea and vomiting in children under 5 take the approach of classifying children into 'no clinically detectable

Box 7.3 Classification into normal, clinical dehydration and shocked (adapted from NICE 2012)

Normal

No clinically detectable dehydration (<5% dehydrated)	No IV fluids needed
No signs of clinical dehydration or shock	Encourage oral fluid intake Offer oral rehydration salts solution to supplement normal fluid intake in high-risk groups (e.g. children younger than 1 year)

Clinical dehydration

Signs of clinical dehydration (5% dehydrated)	Trial of oral or NG replacement Replacement IV fluid (if oral replacement not tolerated/possible)
■ Reduced urine output ■ Sunken eyes ■ Dry mucous membranes ■ Reduced skin turgor ■ Altered behaviour (e.g. lethargic, irritable)	1. Give 50 mL/kg fluid in addition to maintenance fluid volume (Dioralyte if giving NG/oral, 0.9% saline with 5% Dextrose if giving IV) **OR** 2. 'MAINTENANCE PLUS 5%'

Shock

Signs of clinical shock (10% dehydrated)	Replacement IV fluid needed
■ Mottled or pale skin ■ CAPILLARY REFILL TIME >2 sec ■ Cold extremities ■ Tachycardia ■ Tachypnoea ■ Weak peripheral pulses ■ Decreased consciousness level ■ Hypotension (indicates DECOMPENSATED SHOCK)	1. Give 20 mL/kg bolus of 0.9% saline, then add 100 mL/kg to maintenance fluids **OR** 2. Give 20 mL/kg bolus of 0.9% saline, then prescribe 'Maintenance plus 10%'

Call for help early if a child is showing any of the above signs of shock and move to resuscitation area

IV, intravenous; NG, nasogastric.

Box 7.4 Worked examples

Example 1

An 8-year-old girl comes to the emergency department with diarrhoea and vomiting. Her mouth looks dry and her mother tells you that she hasn't passed urine for about 6 h. Her observations and CAPILLARY REFILL TIME are normal, her hands feel warm and she is alert. You don't have a recent weight for this child but based on your clinical findings, you feel that she is 'clinically dehydrated' or 5% dehydrated (see Box 7.3). Her weight today is 25.6 kg.

Method 1

The child is clinically dehydrated and therefore requires 50 mL/kg of additional fluid. This replacement fluid can be given either orally (over 4 h) or IV (over 24 h) in addition to the maintenance fluid requirements over 24 h.

- Maintenance: 100 mL/kg × 10 kg + 50 mL/kg × 10 kg + 20 mL/kg × 5.6 kg = 1612 mL
- Replacement: 50 mL/kg × 25.6 kg = 1280 mL

For oral route: replacement fluid given over 4 h → 1280/4 = 320 mL/h
This is in addition to maintenance requirements 1612/24 = 67 mL/h
Therefore total hourly rate for first 4 h is 320 + 67 = 387 mL/h
387/6 = 65 mL every 10 min
After that, fluid can be given at maintenance rate = 67 mL/h = 11 mL every 10 min or a larger volume, less frequently.
For the IV route, replacement fluid is given over 24 h.
Total in 24 h = Maintenance + Replacement = 1612 + 1280 = 2892 mL
Therefore rate for IV fluids = 2892 mL/24 h = 121 mL/h *but reassess this every 2–4 h.*

Method 2

You estimate that the child is 5% dehydrated based on clinical findings.
Maintenance: 100 mL/kg × 10 kg + 50 mL/kg × 10 kg + 20 mL/kg × 5.6 kg = 1612 mL
Replacement: 5% dehydrated means you estimate that she has lost 5% of her body weight. You know that 1 g body weight is equivalent to 1 mL fluid.
She weighs 25.6 kg so 5% of her body weight = 5/100 × 25.6 = 1.28 kg = 1280 g.
She has lost 1280 g, therefore she will need 1280 mL of additional fluid over 24 h.
Then calculate hourly correction rates for oral or IV options as for the example above.

Example 2

A 6-month-old baby is brought in with a history of diarrhoea and vomiting and his parents say he has been sleepy. On examination, he has a capillary refill

(Continued)

time of 3 sec and has cold hands and feet. In his 'red book' there is a recording of his weight from last week when he visited the GP for his vaccinations; he weighed 6178 g. Today he weighs 5.58 kg so he has lost 598 g.

Method 1

The baby has signs of clinical shock and therefore needs a 20 mL/kg bolus of normal saline and 100 mL/kg of additional fluid.

Fluid bolus (stat fluids): 20 mL/kg × 5.58 kg = 111.6 mL stat of 0.9% saline (it makes sense to round this up to 115 mL stat of 0.9% saline for ease of measuring)

Maintenance: 100 mL/kg × 5.58 kg = 558 mL

Replacement: 100 mL/kg × 5.58 kg = 558 mL

Total over 24 h: 558 mL + 558 mL = 1116 mL

Rate of infusion = 1116 mL/24 h = 46.5 mL/h then round up to 47 mL/h

Method 2

The child is shocked and therefore needs 20 mL/mg bolus of normal saline. You estimate that the child is 10% dehydrated based on clinical findings but you know the *actual* weight loss so can base your calculations on this.

Fluid bolus (stat fluids): 20 mL/kg × 5.58 kg = 111.6 mL stat of 0.9% saline (it makes sense to round this up to 115 mL stat of 0.9% saline for ease of measuring)

Maintenance: 100 mL/kg × 5.58 kg = 558 mL

Replacement: the child has lost 598 g. You know that 1 g weight loss is equivalent to 1 mL of fluid loss therefore he needs 598 mL replacement fluid

Total over 24 h: Maintenance + Replacement = 558 + 598 = 1156 mL

Rate of infusion = 1156 mL/24 h = 48.2 mL/h and then round to 48 mL/h

GP, general practitioner; IV, intravenous.

dehydration', 'clinically dehydrated' or 'shocked' and prescribing a fixed mL/kg volume of additional fluid for each category (see Box 7.3). You may find it easier to remember these volumes if you don't like working through the calculations from first principles. These categories are equivalent to <5%, 5% and 10% dehydrated respectively and the volume of replacement fluid needed works out the same regardless of which of the two methods you use (Box 7.4

Example 1). Using a child's *actual* weight loss (if available) will give you a slightly different, more accurate number (see Box 7.4, Example 2).

Analgesia

Pain relief is extremely important and should not be limited to pharmaceutical intervention alone; anxiety and emotional responses to pain must also be considered. Play specialists are very skilled at distraction techniques to reduce perception of pain and also to alleviate anxiety – make good use of them, particularly when you are the source of the child's pain (e.g. procedures or diagnostics). In infants, sucrose solutions (such as Sweet-Ease or TootSweet) or breast-feeding prior to and during painful procedures can reduce distress.

Topical analgesia such as local anaesthetic cream (e.g. Emla or Ametop) prior to minor practical procedures is also very useful and should always be used unless you have good reasons not to. Apply the cream to the relevant area with a clear adhesive dressing over the top to keep it from rubbing off. It takes 30–60 min to take effect, after which time, remove the dressing and clean off the cream. The skin should be numb where the cream has been and therefore any procedure significantly less painful. In situations where you need to do a procedure as a matter of urgency, a cold spray (such as ethylchloride spray) can be used to numb the area (spray on from 30 cm away for 2–3 sec just before you put needle to skin).

The World Health Organization analgesic ladder should guide your prescription of analgesia with new medications added in a stepwise approach. Assess the severity of the child's pain to guide you as to which step to start at.

Step 1 – mild pain

Paracetamol

Paracetamol should be the mainstay of basic analgesia. It has a good side-effect profile and gives effective pain relief when used in addition to stronger analgesics. It works best when given regularly and also has a useful antipyretic effect. Oral and IV doses are the same. Rectal doses differ so check the BNFc if prescribing rectal paracetamol.

A safe basic dose for all ages either IV or oral is 15 mg/kg up to a maximum of 1 g qds. However, the BNFc recently changed paracetamol doses to giving by age rather than weight so check your dose falls within these ranges. Can be given every 4–6 h, up to a maximum of four times in 24 h.

Non-steroidal anti-inflammatories

Non-steroidal anti-inflammatories (NSAIDs) can be added for mild pain where paracetamol alone is insufficient. NSAIDs work well in combination with paracetamol as they work synergistically to improve the analgesic effect. Ibuprofen has one of the best side-effect profiles of the NSAIDs and is most commonly used. It should preferably be given after food to minimise risk of gastric side-effects. Like paracetamol, ibuprofen also has a useful antipyretic effect.

For children older than 1 month, a basic dose of 5 mg/kg orally is the standard but up to 10 mg/kg can be given. This is also listed in the BNFc by age bracket so check your dose fits these ranges. Can be given every 8 h, up to a maximum of three times daily.

Step 2 – moderate pain

Mild opioids

Codeine phosphate can be given for moderate pain in addition to paracetamol and ibuprofen. It is notorious for causing constipation and it is probably worth prescribing prophylactic laxatives to avoid this.

■ In the over-12s: 30–60mg qds

Dihydrocodeine has a similar profile to codeine phosphate. It is licensed for use in children over 4 years.

■ Child 4–12 years: 0.5–1mg/kg (max 30mg) every 4–6 hours

■ Child over 12: 30mg every 4–6 hours

Step 3 – severe pain

Strong opioids

For severe pain, stronger opioids can be given alongside Step 1 analgesia and **instead of mild opioids**.

Morphine is the most commonly used strong opiate. It comes in many different preparations (oral solution, tablets, injection, modified and immediate release); choose the most appropriate for optimising concordance and rapidity of onset of analgesia required. Doses for oral solution.

■ For children 6 months–12 years: 200 micrograms/kg up to every 4h as needed (max 10mg)

■ For children over 12 years: 5–10mg up to every 4h as needed

The key for strong opiates is to titrate the dose to the child's pain. Start with a smaller dose and gradually increase if necessary. Always monitor for signs of reduced respiratory rate or reduced level of consciousness.

Controlled drugs

Controlled drugs must be prescribed in a certain way if they are to be given as a prescription to take home. Commonly prescribed controlled drugs include strong opioids and benzodiazepines.

When prescribing a controlled drug, there are certain things which must be present on the prescription.

■ Name and address of the patient

■ The form and strength of preparation (e.g. morphine oral solution 10mg/5mL)

■ The total quantity or number of dose units in both words and figures (e.g. 50mL fifty millilitres in total or 10 ten tablets in total)

■ The dose and frequency (e.g. 10mg as required, maximum of every 4h)

■ Signed and dated by the prescriber and specify prescriber's address (hospital or GP practice)

Blood products

When prescribing blood products in children, it is important to first consider if they have any special requirements such as cytomegalovirus (CMV) negative or irradiated products. Below are examples of situations in which these are needed but if in any doubt, check with a senior paediatrician and check the patient's medical records. See the Transfusion Handbook at www.transfusionguidelines.org for more details.

When to give CMV-negative products

Cytomegalovirus can cause serious pathology in immunocompromised patients who have never previously been exposed to it. Patients who need CMV-negative blood products include:

■ children who have had allogenic stem cell grafts and who are CMV negative

■ children with HIV

■ intrauterine transfusions

■ all children under 1 year of age.

When to give gamma-irradiated products

Irradiated products are given to immunocompromised patients who are at risk of transfusion-associated graft-versus-host disease, which is a potentially fatal complication of transfusion and therefore irradiated products must be given to all those at risk. These include:

■ children with Hodgkin's disease

■ children taking chemotherapy/immunosuppressants (e.g. methotrexate)

■ children with congenital immunodeficiency (e.g. severe combined immunodeficiency [SCID], Di George syndrome)

■ children who have had bone marrow transplants

■ intrauterine transfusions

■ rxchange transfusions.

Packed red cells

In children, red cells are prescribed by volume in millilitres, *not* units. Volume required is calculated using the formula:

(Target haemoglobin

– actual haemoglobin) × weight in kg × 3

= red cell volume to prescribe

The recommended rate of transfusion is 5 mL/kg/h for standard transfusion. Red cells may need to be administered more rapidly in major haemorrhage. Maximum time from removal of red cells from fridge to completion of transfusion is 4 h.

Volume and rate of infusion of red cells in NEONATES vary with indication – see 'Transfusion of the Newborn Infant' in the Transfusion Handbook at www.transfusionguidelines.org for details.

> ### Ethical Dilemma
>
> Receiving blood transfusions is against the religious beliefs of Jehovah's Witnesses. This can be very difficult when faced with a child who requires a blood transfusion whose parents are refusing to give consent for this. In the event of blood transfusion being a life-saving emergency treatment (e.g. in major haemorrhage), transfusion can be given without the consent of the child's parents. In non-emergency situations, if it is absolutely necessary that the child has a blood transfusion, permission can be sought through the courts for you to go ahead with transfusion against the parents' wishes.

Platelets

For infants and children who weigh over 15 kg, platelets are prescribed in units (~300 mL volume). For children under 15 kg, platelets are given at a volume of 10–20 mL/kg.

Platelets are infused at a rate of 10–20 mL/kg/h.

Fresh frozen plasma (FFP)

Volume of FFP is 10–20 mL/kg, given at a rate of 10–20 mL/kg/h.

Drug level monitoring

Some drugs require monitoring of serum levels in order to adjust the dose administered accordingly. This may be because they have a narrow therapeutic window or are particularly toxic at high levels. The levels need to be taken at a time when you would expect the blood concentrations of the blood to have reached a steady state. Some examples of drug which require serum monitoring and when you should take the sample are listed in Table 7.1. *Local policy on dosing and levels may vary – check your local protocols or with your ward pharmacist.*

Table 7.1 Some examples of drugs that require serum monitoring

Drug name	When to take the first blood sample	Normal therapeutic range
Aminophylline/ theophylline	**Oral**: 5 days after starting treatment, 'trough' level 8 h post dose or immediately predose **IV**: 4–6 h after starting treatment. If already on oral theophylline, do not give loading dose of IV aminophylline. Ideally take levels before starting infusion but do not delay treatment waiting for results in life-threatening asthma	**Acute severe asthma**: 10–20 mg/litre **Neonatal apnoea**: 8–12 mg/litre
Digoxin	Measure 7 days after starting oral dose at least 6 h post dose Measure 4 h after IV dose	0.8–2 micrograms/litre
Gentamicin	**Multiple daily dose regime**: 1 h post dose 'peak' level Predose 'trough' level	5–10 mg/litre 3–5 mg/litre for endocarditis 8–12 mg/litre in cystic fibrosis <2 mg/litre <1 mg/litre for endocarditis
	Once-daily regime: predose 'trough' level (usually taken prior to the 2nd or 3rd dose)	<1 mg/litre

Table 7.1 (cont'd)

Drug name	When to take the first blood sample	Normal therapeutic range
Phenobarbital	Measure 2 weeks after starting oral treatment. Take 'trough' blood sample 8 h post dose or immediately predose	15–40 mg/litre
Phenytoin	Take sample 2 h after IV loading dose	Neonate–3 months: 6–15 mg/litre
	Take sample 2 weeks after starting oral treatment. Take 'trough' level 8 h post dose or immediately predose	Child 3 months–18 years: 10–20 mg/litre. After IV loading dose, if level 10–20 mg/L; start maintenance. If <10 mg/L give a further loading dose of 5 mg/kg
Vancomycin	Take predose 'trough' blood sample (usually taken before giving the 3rd dose)	5–15 mg/litre 5–10 mg/litre in renal impairment

IV, intravenous

Useful websites

BNFc: for the online version of the BNFc visit http://bnfc.org/bnfc/index.htm

Prescribing practice: get some practice prescribing from our additional materials provided at www.wileyhandsonguides.com/paediatrics

Further prescribing practice available at: http:// www.rcpch.ac.uk/training-examinations-professional-development/quality-training/paediatric-prescribing-tool/paediatr

Drug information for parents and patients: www.medicinesforchildren.org.uk/

Medicines for Children Research Network: www.mcrn.org.uk

Reference

National Institute for Health and Clinical Excellence (2012) *Diarrhoea and Vomiting in Children Under 5: Quick Reference Guide*. NICE Guideline No. CG84. National Institute for Health and Clinical Excellence, London

Chapter 8
TEENAGERS

The teenage years involve many physical, emotional and cognitive changes. Whilst many teenagers will make the transition to adulthood relatively straightforwardly, for others it can be a stressful and difficult time.

Taking a history from a teenager

Some suggestions for how to communicate effectively with teenagers are outlined in Chapter 3 – Communication.

It is important to be aware of your communication style whilst taking a history from a teenager but in addition to style, you also need to think about the content of your history. For example, asking a birth history is unlikely to be relevant for a teenager but there are other issues that are likely to be important in this age group.

The following are important to discuss when taking a history from a teenager:

■ **Confidentiality**. In order to allow the young person to feel comfortable in sharing information with you, it is helpful to remind them that any information they share with you will remain confidential (unless you have significant concerns for their own, or other people's, safety in which case you will share the relevant information with only the necessary people). *For more information about confidentiality, consent and consultation style, see Chapter 3 – Communication.*

■ **Home**. Where do they live? Who do they live with? How are things at home? Do they have any difficult relationships with people at home?

■ **Education**. Are they still at school or at a college or working? What school/college do they go to or where do they work? Do they enjoy it? How are they finding the school work/exams/working environment? Who are their friends? Are they being bullied?

■ **Activities**. What do they do when they are not at school or work? Are they part of a gang? Do they attend any youth groups or organisations?

■ **Drugs, smoking and alcohol**. This can be a difficult one to ask about. You may find it helpful to ask about their friends first: 'some people your age will drink alcohol, is that something that your friends do? Then after they have answered this, you can go on to ask if they also consume alcohol. You need to

The Hands-on Guide to Practical Paediatrics, First Edition. Rebecca Hewitson and Caroline Fertleman.
© 2014 John Wiley & Sons, Ltd. Published 2014 by John Wiley & Sons, Ltd.
Companion Website: www.wileyhandsonguides.com/paediatrics

find out exactly what, how much and how frequently they consume drugs, alcohol or cigarettes. If you don't know the slang name for a street drug, clarify with them what they mean but avoid using slang yourself if they are not. With alcohol, you can also ask if they feel that their drinking ever gets out of control or they think that they drink too much.

■ **Diet**. Ask about eating habits and if they have any concerns about their weight or the way that their body looks?

■ **Sex**. Do they have a boyfriend or girl-friend? Are they having sex? Are they using contraception and practising safe sex? Do they have any problems or wor-ries about anything relating to sex? *See the Sexual health section below for more details.*

■ **Mental health**. How are they feel-ing? Low mood? Anxious? How are they

 Top Tip

In most circumstances it is inappropriate to ask a young person about their sexual health or substance use in front of their parents. This can be extremely embarrassing for them, is very unlikely to yield any honest answers and may undermine their trust in you. Always allow time for a young person to see you on their own and bring up these topics at this stage. Reminding them that the consultation is confidential and that you will not share any information with anyone without asking the young person's permission can be very helpful in encouraging them to talk to you.

sleeping? Any suicidal thoughts or attempts at taking their own life? *See the Mental health section below for more details.*

Mental health problems

Much of the specialist management for children and young people with mental health problems is delivered or super-vised by the Child and Adolescent Mental Health team. However, it is important for all doctors working with children and young people to know how to manage acute mental health problems and their accompanying medical signs and symptoms.

A useful website for young people and their parents about mental health issues is Young Minds (www.youngminds.org.uk).

Deliberate self-harm and suicide

Deliberate self-harm is common and frequently dealt with in the emergency department. Suicidal intent is not the only reason for self-harm, although a small proportion of those who self-harm will go on to commit suicide.

Self-harm is frequently an impulsive act that may follow an argument or upsetting situation. It can be a cry for help, a physical way of relieving emo-tional distress, a way to 'get back at' other people or a suicide attempt. All self-harm must be taken seriously as, even if the child does not appear at risk of suicide, it is an indication of severe emotional distress.

When caring for a child who is presenting following self-harm or attempted suicide:

■ **Deal with any medical problems**. It is important to immediately establish any medical or surgical problems from a brief history and examination and to initiate appropriate treatment. You may need to involve the surgical team for help with suturing deep wounds (remembering to always use appropriate analgesia). *For emergency management of overdose, drowning and Basic Life Support, see Chapter 5 – Common Paediatric Emergencies.*

■ **Keep the child or young person safe**. Until you have had time to take a history and establish any ongoing risk of self-harm, it is important not to leave the patient unsupervised.

■ **Assess ongoing risk**. You need to establish the level of ongoing risk of the patient completing a further episode of self-harm. This will help to inform your decision about the most appropriate management plan. *See Box 8.1 for risk and protective factors for ongoing risk of self-harm or suicide.*

■ **Ask about suicidal thoughts**. This can be difficult to ask about but starting with a generalised statement may help, such as: 'Some young people tell me that they sometimes feel that life is not worth living; have you ever felt like that?'.

■ **Find out about plans**. 'Have you ever made plans about how you might end your life? Have you ever started trying to follow through with those plans?'

■ **Perform a brief mental state examination**. This will be done in more detail by the mental health team but is important to undertake this at the time of presentation. Document:

– **appearance and behaviour**. Are they behaving normally and communicating with you? Do they appear unkempt or smartly dressed? How do you think they appear – sad, inappropriately cheerful, agitated?

– **speech**. Very quiet and withdrawn? Few words at all? Loud and pressured speech?

Box 8.1   Risk and protective factors for repeated self-harm or attempted suicide

For any child or young person presenting with self-harm or attempted suicide, it is crucial to assess their ongoing risk to themselves. It is important to ask a detailed history in a sensitive way to establish any concerning features that may suggest that the young person is at risk of repeated self-harm, and also potential sources of support.

Risk factors for repeat self-harm or suicide

Worrying features of this episode

- Conducted in isolation
- Precautions taken to avoid discovery
- Planned rather than impulsive
- Suicide note or message
- Did not ask for help during or after act
- Violent method – firearms, hanging, jumping off high place or into traffic

Personal risk factors

- Known mental health problems
- Previous self-harm or suicide attempts
- Low self-esteem
- Use of alcohol or drugs (increase impulsive behaviour)

Social risk factors or triggers

- Poor relationship with family
- Victim of abuse or neglect
- Bereavement
- Break-up or argument with close friend or boyfriend/girlfriend
- Parents with substance misuse
- Parents with mental health problems
- Isolation
- Easy access to the means of self-harm

Reassuring factors in history

- Patient regrets having self-harmed
- No ongoing plans to attempt suicide or to self-harm
- Supportive family and friends
- Willingness to engage with services providing support

– **mood**. Ask the young person how they are feeling. It can be helpful to record their response verbatim.

– **unusual beliefs or hallucinations**. Do they appear to have any delusional belief or hallucinations?

– **insight**. Do they understand what the problem is and why they are in hospital?

■ **Admit to the ward**. The safest approach for all cases of children presenting following an episode of self-harm is to arrange inpatient admission. This will allow monitoring of their medical condition and also will ensure their safety whilst awaiting assessment and input from the CHILD AND ADOLESCENT MENTAL HEALTH SERVICE (CAMHS). Following your risk assessment, you may feel that the child is safe to be admitted to a normal paediatric ward, or that they will need one-to-one nursing, or that they need admission to a specialist mental health unit.

■ **Discuss with your seniors**. It is very important to inform your registrar or the consultant on call about any child or young person presenting with self-harm and ensure that they are happy with your proposed management plan.

■ **liaise with camhs and children's social care**. It is important for all children and young people presenting with self-harm to have input from the CAMHS team. It may also be appropriate to involve social services to find out more about the child's social circumstances (to identify both protective and risk factors for further episodes of self-harm).

Eating disorders

It is unusual for a young person to present with an eating disorder. They may well present with other symptoms or signs that have resulted from their eating disorder (such as their menstrual periods having stopped or feeling fatigued) or they may be brought in by a parent who is concerned about their eating habits.

This can be a very difficult subject to broach and many young people may be secretive about exactly how much they are eating and drinking and try to conceal their illness from others.

There are some dangerous medical complications of anorexia and bulimia that need to be considered in your management of these patients. Assessment of various parameters in the history, examination and investigations can help to assess the level of risk of such complications occurring.

When seeing a patient with an eating disorder check the following.

■ **How much are they actually eating and drinking?** Severe restriction of intake (to less than 50% of expected), restriction of fluid intake, vomiting or the use of laxatives are all concerning features.

■ **Heart rate and rhythm**. Bradycardia is a concerning sign; be particularly worried about a heart rate lower than 50 beats per minute. Arrhythmias are also a worrying sign; take an electrocardiogram (ECG) to look for irregularity or prolonged QT interval.

■ **Blood pressure**. This may present itself as a history of recurrent fainting.

Marked postural drop (>15 mmHg systolic) is a very worrying sign.

■ **Hydration**. Check for signs of dehydration as in severe cases patients may have stopped drinking as well as eating.

■ **Temperature**. A temperature of <36°C is a worrying sign.

■ **Check electrolytes and albumin**. Patients who are restricting their oral intake can have very low serum electrolyte and albumin levels. Check for phosphate, potassium, sodium, calcium and albumin. Low levels of any of these is a worrying sign and the patient must be monitored very closely for refeeding syndrome once oral intake is restarted.

■ **Do they have any insight?** Do they recognise that there is a problem with their eating? Are they motivated to change their behaviour?

■ **Are they exercising excessively?** Some patients will exercise for over an hour a day in addition to restricting their oral intake.

■ **Are they at risk of self-harm or suicide?** Patients with eating disorders are at increased risk of self-harm or suicide. They are also more likely to have concurrent illnesses such as obsessive compulsive disorder.

Your initial assessment of these parameters is important for making decisions about where the patient will be best managed (usually only those who are clinically unstable require hospital admission). Always involve your senior colleagues, a dietitian and the CAMHS team in management of these patients.

Organisations which may be helpful for patients and their parents about eating disorders include Beat (www.b-eat.co.uk) and Body Gossip, a positive body image campaign (www.bodygossip.org).

Substance abuse

It is important to ask all teenagers about alcohol, tobacco and illicit drug use as part of your routine history taking. By the age of 15 years, 45% of UK adolescents will have drunk alcohol, 25% will have tried smoking and 30% will have tried cannabis.

Certain degrees of experimentation and risk taking form a normal part of teenage behaviour. However, in teenagers for whom you suspect that their alcohol or drug use is out of their control or becoming a concern, it is important to consider both the causes and the consequences of their behaviour. Do they have an underlying anxiety disorder or depression? Are they living in difficult social circumstances? Have they previously been or are currently subject to abuse? You also need to consider the result of their substance misuse as drug and alcohol use can lead to more impulsive behaviour. This can put young people at increased risk of unwanted pregnancy or sexually transmitted diseases through unsafe sex, can be associated with deliberate self-harm and may even put others at risk as well as themselves (for example, if driving whilst intoxicated).

When asking about substance misus, use the following questions.

■ **What are they using?** This includes alcohol and tobacco as well as street drugs. Do not use slang names yourself and clarify any language used by the young person that you are not familiar with.

■ **How much and how often?** You need to find out how frequently they are consuming alcohol/tobacco/drugs and how much.

■ **Ever had too much?** Ask about drinking to excess and need for hospital attendance or overdose of drugs. *For specific details about the signs, symptoms and management of overdose with different substances, see the Overdose section of Chapter 5 – Common Paediatric Emergencies.*

■ **Dependence**. Do they have difficulty controlling their use? Do they need to use more now than they used to in order to get the same effect? Do they have any withdrawal symptoms?

■ **Impact on their life**. Warning signs that there may be a problem tend to be relatively non-specific such as a drop in school results, violence, theft or isolation.

The CRAFFT questions can be helpful for assessing risk taking behaviour. A copy of this questionnaire is available to download from http://www.ceasar-boston.org/CRAFFT/.

FRANK is a website that has lots of useful information about drugs for young people and parents, including a free phone hotline, online chats and email service. It also has a slang dictionary for different drug names which may be useful for professionals (www.talktofrank.com).

Sexual health

This is a topic that most people (patients and doctors alike) find difficult to talk about, but it is a particularly important one to get right.

Here are some suggestions for how to take a good sexual history.

■ **Ask routinely**. Taking a sexual history will become easier the more you practise. Try to make a brief sexual history a routine part of all consultations with teenagers.

■ **Ask permission**. Before asking questions about sexuality, it may be helpful to give some warning and to ask the young person if this is OK, such as 'I'd like to ask you some more personal questions now that I ask all of my patients your age. I won't tell other people about what we discuss (unless I'm worried that you or someone else is in serious danger) and you don't have to answer all the questions if you feel uncomfortable. Would that be OK?'.

■ **Acknowledge embarrassment**. If a young person appears obviously fearful or embarrassed then it may be helpful to acknowledge that many people find talking about sex very difficult and embarrassing and that they are courageous for talking to you about it.

■ **Be matter of fact**. Try to be as unembarrassed as possible yourself as this will help the young person to relax and talk about this difficult topic. Generalisations can make difficult questions easier to ask; for example, 'Many people your age will be starting to think about having sex, is that the case for you?'.

■ **Be non-judgemental**. Make sure that you are aware of your facial expressions and body language whilst you are listening. Frowning, showing surprise or disgust, crossing your arms or avoiding eye contact can all discourage the patient from continuing to talk as they may interpret these as you passing judgement on what they are saying.

■ **Avoid jargon and slang**. Avoid using medical jargon when talking to patients about sex and sexuality but also do not use slang terms as this can be alarming, offensive or patronising; young people expect their doctors to be professionals. Use plain, simple language.

■ **Don't make assumptions**. This involves assumptions about the young person's level of understanding or experience, who they are having sex with and what kind of sex and why they have come to see you. Ask questions in an open-ended way that avoids implied assumptions or criticisms.

■ **Let them ask you questions**. Many young people will have lots of anxieties and uncertainties about sex and taking a sexual history can provide a valuable opportunity for them to gain information from you. Some may be too shy to ask and generalisations can again be useful here, such as: 'Many young people have worries or questions about sex or their bodies. Would you like to ask me some questions about anything?'.

■ **Be alert for signs of abuse**. It is important to always consider the possibility that a young person has been coerced or forced into taking part in sexual activities. Always consider the possibility of sexual abuse, forced marriage, sex trafficking and FEMALE GENITAL MUTILATION. Much sexual abuse and harassment of young people is perpetrated by their peers, but having an older partner is a significant risk factor. *See Chapter 4 – Child Protection and Safeguarding for details on concerning teenage sexual behaviour, forced marriage and female genital mutilation.*

Brook is a charity that provides sexual health clinics and advice for young people under 25. Its website (www.brook.org.uk) has lots of useful information for patients and professionals and there is a free confidential helpline for patients.

TheSite.org (www.thesite.org) has lots of advice for teenagers about sex and relationships, health, drugs and alcohol, amongst other things.

Chapter 9
NEONATES

Perhaps the most daunting of all for those starting out in paediatrics is the alien world of the NEONATE; they're so tiny and yet so terrifying. A reassuring word from a neonatal consultant: 'It helps to remember, these creatures are tough and built to survive'. It also helps to remember that you should have a low threshold for calling in reinforcements and no one will criticise you for doing so.

The term 'neonate' is used for babies who are less than 4 weeks old and 'infant' is normally used to describe any baby who is less than 1 year.

Neonatal life support at birth

See the newborn life support algorithm (Fig. 9.1).

Make sure you familiarise yourself with the RESUSCITAIRES at your hospital before you are first called to a delivery. Put on gloves and apron as soon as you arrive so that you're ready. Whilst you are waiting for the obstetricians to do their bit, check that all your equipment is available and working (Box 9.1).

Understanding the basic physiology of the immediate postnatal period may help you to remember what you should be doing and why. For a good explanation which is quick and easy to read, look at the 'Newborn Life Support' section of the resuscitation guidelines at www.resus.org.uk.

Key points are as follows.

1 Get the baby dry and keep them warm – babies can lose heat very quickly.

2 Make sure they are adequately aerating their lungs and support their airway and/or breathing in order to achieve this if necessary.

3 Slow heart rate is almost always a reflection of not having achieved adequate ventilation and will normally improve once you have managed this.

4 Call for help early.

The following steps apply to the resuscitation of term babies. For variations required when resuscitating preterm infants, see the 'Prematurity' section below.

Once the baby is out:

■ start timer

■ don't drop them (use a towel if being passed to you – they're very slippery when you have gloves on)

The Hands-on Guide to Practical Paediatrics, First Edition. Rebecca Hewitson and Caroline Fertleman.
© 2014 John Wiley & Sons, Ltd. Published 2014 by John Wiley & Sons, Ltd.
Companion Website: www.wileyhandsonguides.com/paediatrics

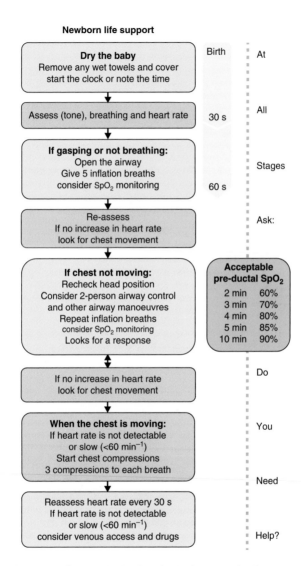

Figure 9.1 Newborn life support algorithm. Reproduced with permission from Resuscitation Council UK.

Box 9.1   Checking the RESUSCITAIRE

Whilst you are doing this, listen out for noises (or a baby crying) to indicate that the baby is out and you need to start the timer.

■ At least two clean, dry towels should be laid out on the Resuscitaire.

■ Turn on the heater (usually to a 'prewarm' setting) to start warming the towels.

■ Turn on the overhead light on the Resuscitaire.

■ Check that there is a stethoscope on the Resuscitaire or you have your own with you.

■ Check that oxygen and air supplies are attached at the wall or to cylinders at the back.

■ Make sure the air-oxygen 'blender' is initially set to 21% oxygen, i.e. air only.

■ Check masks of appropriate size are available (e.g. if baby is known to be preterm, get smaller masks out).

■ Check the inflation pressure is set to roughly 30 cmH_2O (or 20–25 cmH_2O for preterms). You can test this by taking the mask off and occluding the end of the T-piece with your hand before inflating (Fig. 9.2).

■ Attach the Yankauer sucker (see Fig. 9.2) to suction and check it is working by obscuring the end (you should see the pressure gauge rise).

■ Check the oxygen saturation monitor is available and the sensor is connected to the machine.

■ Check that you have the appropriate laryngoscopes (one long and one short blade) and that they are both lighting up properly when opened.

■ Check that tracheal tubes are available on the Resuscitaire for rare cases when the baby requires intubation (by someone experienced).

■ Check you have oropharyngeal (GUEDEL) AIRWAYS available. Again, check that you have several sizes but you can usually anticipate likely size.

If you've arrived in plenty of time then you may also want to check through the antenatal and birth notes for any issues during antenatal testing or labour which you should be aware of or ask the midwife. Particular concerns are risk factors for sepsis or anomalies identified on the scan.

■ dry vigorously and discard wet towel

■ wrap in dry towel

■ assess:

– airway

– breathing

– heart rate

– tone

– colour.

1 Airway patent? Position the baby's head in the neutral position to open the airway (Fig. 9.3). If the airway still remains obviously obstructed, look in the mouth and suction if you can see something obstructing the airway. **Do not suction further down than you can see as you may cause laryngospasm.**

2 Breathing spontaneously? Is the baby crying? If they are screaming you can start relaxing. If not, then assess are they breathing regularly and rapidly?

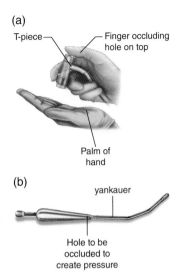

Figure 9.2 *T-piece and Yankauer sucker.*

Can you hear air entry when listening to the chest?

3 Is their heart rate greater than 100 beats per minute?

4 Are their arms and legs flexed? Are they wriggling around?

5 Are they pink? It is normal for babies to be born blue but start to turn pink rapidly after birth. Acrocyanosis (blue/purple hands and feet) is normal even after several minutes but the baby should be pink centrally by this time.

If the answer to any of these questions (particularly breathing and heart rate) is 'no' then you need to do something about it. Try each of the following in turn and reassess using the above questions every 30 sec.

Neonatal life support at birth | **203**

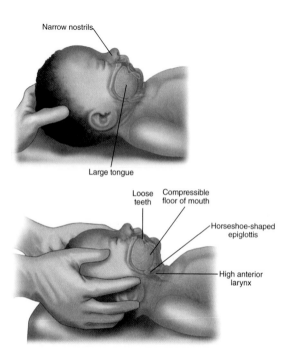

Narrow nostrils

Large tongue

Loose teeth

Compressible floor of mouth

Horseshoe-shaped epiglottis

High anterior larynx

Figure 9.3 Opening the airway of an infant using a head tilt and chin lift. (a) Airway occluded. (b) Airway opened using head tilt and chin lift.

Stimulate and airway manoeuvre

Stimulate by rubbing the back or soles of feet with the towel. To open the airway, you need to bring the baby's head to a neutral position (i.e. so that their face is parallel to the surface on which they are lying). Newborn babies tend to have a prominent occiput which can make achieving this difficult; sometimes placing something under their shoulders can help with this. Be careful not to overextend the neck as this can occlude the airway.

Reassess

Most babies should have established spontaneous breathing by roughly 90 sec of age. If they are still not breathing or the heart rate remains low after stimulation and airway positioning, move to giving inflation breaths. Whilst you are still learning, it can be difficult assessing if breathing is adequate. If you are unsure, it is far better to give the inflation breaths than not.

Give five inflation breaths

Ensure that you have positioned the head so that the airway is open whilst delivering inflation breaths. These inflation breaths should be about 2 sec duration each. Use the T-piece apparatus (which should be available on virtually all RESUSCITAIRES now) (see Fig. 9.2) as it allows you to deliver more accurate pressures and is less cumbersome than the bag and mask. Your eyes need to be on the baby's chest to check that it is moving as you deliver the breaths so to keep track of time count '1 and 2 and 3 and' as you give each breath. This takes about 2 sec even if you're stressed and talking quickly! You can keep track of how many breaths you've given this way too by counting '2 and 2 and 3 and… 3 and 2 and 3 and…' etc. up to 5.

Reassess

If the baby's condition has still not improved at this stage, consider putting out a crash call (if you haven't already) in order to get more help.

Consider oxygen saturation monitoring

Ask for help from whomever is already in the room to put an oxygen saturation probe on whilst you continue to manage the airway. This can give you an objective measure of progress and will also give you the baby's heart rate. Make sure that you *place the probe on the right hand* in order to record PREDUCTAL

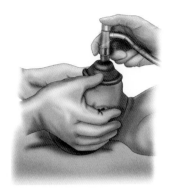

Figure 9.4 Two-person technique for delivering inflation breaths.

readings. Acceptable preductal oxygen saturation levels increase gradually over the first few minutes of life:

- 2 min 60%
- 3 min 70%
- 4 min 80%
- 5 min 85%
- 10 min 90%.

Further inflation breaths or regular breaths

If you have delivered your inflation breaths successfully then you should start to see a rapid increase in the baby's heart rate. If the heart rate remains low then assume that this is because your inflation breaths weren't successful and try again (possibly using the two-person technique, with a jaw thrust, for delivery of breaths to improve chances of success – see Fig. 9.4). Watch carefully to see if the chest rises.

If you are sure that you saw the chest rise when delivering the inflation breaths and/or the baby's heart rate has increased but the baby is not yet breathing spontaneously then continue regular breaths at a rate of 30–40 per minute until the baby establishes spontaneous breathing.

 Top Tip

If in any doubt about the baby's condition, ask someone to put out an arrest call. This will vary between hospitals – some have a dedicated neonatal team with separate bleeps, some don't. Make sure you know what the local policy is so that you know whether to ask for a 'paediatric crash call' or 'neonatal crash call' so that you get the relevant people turning up quickly to help you.

Calculating Apgar scores

Apgar scores are still used as an approximation of how well or otherwise a baby is progressing in the minutes immediately following delivery. Their primary aim is to show how successful resuscitation efforts have been and over what period of time. They are recorded as scores at 1, 5 and 10 min. They are not really used at the time to inform resuscitation decisions but instead are calculated afterwards to give others an idea of the baby's

Apgar score	
Heart rate	
>100	2 points
<100	1 point
Absent	0 points
Respiratory effort	
Crying	2 points
Slow (irregular)	1 point
Absent	0 points
Tone	
Active motion	2 points
Some flexion of extremities	1 point
Limp	0 points
Colour	
All pink	2 points
Pink body, blue extremities	1 point
Pale, blue	0 points
Response to stimulation	
Strong cry	2 points
Weak cry	1 point
No response	0 points

Adapted from Dr Virginia Apgar's original paper published in 1953.

condition and response to resuscitation. The score given to a baby can be a rather subjective measure and the important thing is to see improvement over time. Some labour notes will contain a specific table in which to record the Apgar scores.

Newborn baby checks

This is a screening process to help rule out any clinically detectable abnormalities before the baby is discharged from hospital. It is also an opportunity for parents to ask questions about the baby so be prepared to be asked all sorts of weird and wonderful things. Be honest if you don't know the answer and also bear in mind that for questions about the minutiae of childcare, the answer may well be 'It probably doesn't matter which you choose to do'. It may be helpful to suggest that they refer to a parenting book, such as *Your Baby Week by Week* (Cave and Fertleman 2007), for these kinds of details.

In order to be able to detect abnormalities, you need to know what they look like! A useful website for learning about some of these, with great photos and explanations, is http://newborns.stanford.edu/Residents/Exam.html.

Different hospitals will have different methods of recording outcomes of the baby check. currently an electronic system for recording baby checks (Newborn and Infant Physical Examination Programme) is being piloted at some centres. Make sure that you know how your hospital expects you to record findings of the baby checks. It is also important to know what to do about any abnormalities that you do find. Many hospitals will have guidelines on how and what follow-up to arrange for common findings (e.g. sacral dimple or risk factors for developmental dysplasia of the hips).

See Table 9.1 for common normal and abnormal findings.

At first baby checks can take quite a long time to do but you will soon develop ways of performing them more efficiently. Here are some pointers for what to include.

First of all, check through the maternity notes for any problems you need to be aware of and ask the mother about any problems during pregnancy or delivery. Specific things to look for in the notes and to ask the parents are as follows.

■ At what gestation was baby born?

■ Any anomalies identified on 20-week scan?

■ Down syndrome screening performed? Less than 1 in 150 is defined as low risk (e.g. 1 in 200 is low risk)

■ Maternal antenatal screening blood tests (e.g. rubella, HIV, Hep B, blood group etc.)

■ Maternal Group B strep

■ Maternal diabetes, genital herpes, HIV, Hep B or other chronic conditions

■ Family history of developmental dysplasia of the hip?

■ Family history of congenital heart disease?

■ Family history of any inherited disorders?

■ Baby lying breech in third trimester?

■ Method of delivery?

■ Any social concerns?

Also check in the baby's notes or postnatal notes and ask the parents the following.

Table 9.1 Common findings at newborn checks – normal and not normal.

Organ	Normal finding	Follow-up or senior advice needed
Skin	Dermal melanosis ('blue spots') Erythema toxicum Milia Sebaceous hyperplasia Dry skin	Naevus flammeus (port-wine stain) – can be associated with other abnormalities
Head and skull	Moulding – abnormal shaped skull, resolves spontaneously Fontanelles soft Caput – resolves spontaneously	Small head circumference (50th centile 35 cm) – plot on growth chart along with birth weight, should be on similar CENTILES Cephalohaematoma – at risk of jaundice
Ears		Low-set – if you draw an imaginary line from eyes out around the skull, the ears should cross or touch this line Incomplete folding of helices of the ears
Eyes	Subconjunctival haemorrhage Oedema of eyelids	Conjunctivitis Cataracts
Mouth	Epstein pearls Tongue tie – rarely needs division	Cleft palate
Neck and clavicles	Clavicular fracture	Goitre
Chest	Breast buds (influence of maternal hormones)	Widely spaced nipples
Arms and hands	Symmetrical movements and normal posture of both arms	Syndactyly Polydactyly Single palmar crease
Abdomen	Small liver edge palpable	Spleen palpable Other abdominal mass
Umbilical cord	Dried out Small, reducible umbilical hernia	Discharge, odour or erythema of skin surrounding umbilical cord

Table 9.1 (cont'd)

Organ	Normal finding	Follow-up or senior advice needed
Genitalia	White vaginal discharge Small spots of vaginal blood (pseudomenses) Patent anus, normal position and size	Hydrocoele – GP follow-up to ensure resolution One undescended testicle – GP follow-up to ensure resolution Bilateral undescended testes – check carefully for other signs of ambiguous genitalia, needs senior review and abdominal ultrasound Hypospadias – warn parents child must not be circumcised
Legs and feet	Both femoral pulses palpable	Talipes equinovarus (club foot) Syndactyly Polydactyly Dislocatable hips (pressure on flexed knees to push hip posteriorly out of joint) or dislocated hips (clunk of hip back into joint on abduction of hips) – needs urgent referral
Back and spine	Small shallow dimple (can see the base) in midline in gluteal crease with no associated skin changes Dermal melanosis over buttocks	Prominent tuft of hair over sacral spine Deep dimple over sacral spine
Reflexes	Moro reflex – should have symmetrical movement of both arms	

GP, general practitioner.

■ Required resuscitation at birth?

■ Apgar scores at delivery?

■ Vitamin K given? If yes, was it intra-muscular or oral? (If given orally then the baby will need to be given two further oral doses – you may be responsible for arranging this or making the GP aware)

■ Method of feeding and is the baby feeding well?

■ Has the baby passed urine and meconium within first 24 h?

■ If observations have been done for the baby, are they normal?

 Top Tip

It can be almost impossible to perform certain parts of the baby check examination if the baby is screaming and unsettled (not to mention pretty uncomfortable on your ears and stressful for the parents). Some pointers may help.

■ Offering your own gloved finger or a parent's little finger for the baby to suck on can create peace and quiet (whilst simultaneously checking their palate and suck reflex).

■ Some bits of the baby check (e.g. head circumference, checking the scalp, red reflex) can be done whilst the parents are cuddling baby.

■ If you're really not getting anywhere, it may be quicker and less stressful for everyone to come back just after the baby has fed when they will be sleepy and more relaxed.

Newborn examination

It can be helpful to do this in an opportunistic way, i.e. first doing the bits that require a baby who is quiet rather than screaming

First of all, just observe that the baby is making symmetrical movements, has normal facial features and is pink in colour. Do they look jaundiced or pale? Are they moving one arm much less than the other? Do they have unusual (DYSMORPHIC) facial features?

As you are handling the baby, notice whether they have good tone and that they are not floppy, but remember that they are unable to support their own head and you will need to do this for them.

Listen to the chest anteriorly for heart and lung sounds, ensuring that the heart sounds are louder on the left than the right and that you cannot hear any murmurs. Look for signs of respiratory distress.

Measure oxygen saturations in the right hand and in one of the feet (reflecting both the pre- and postductal circulation). Saturations should be above 96% and within 2% of one another.

Check red reflexes in both eyes. Turning off the lights in the room to do this will often encourage babies to open their eyes and enable you to see the red reflex more clearly.

Once you've managed to get these key 'quiet baby' things done first, the baby needs a full top-to-toe examination.

Prematurity

Prematurity is defined as any baby born at less than 37 weeks' gestation. However, the extent to which babies require additional care and have long-term health problems as a result varies enormously with gestational age. Babies born between 34 and 36 weeks' gestation are considered 'late preterms', whilst those born at less than 28 weeks are 'extremely preterm' with below 25 weeks' gestation being considered at the 'borderline of viability'.

The birth weight of the baby also plays an important part in prognosis. Prematurity is not always the underlying reason for low birth weight – a baby may be small for gestational age. Birth weight for *term babies* is normally con-sidered to be classified around the ranges in the following box.

Normal birth weight	2500–4000 g
Low birth weight	<2500 g
Very low birth weight	<1500 g
Extremely low birth weight	<1000 g

Babies whose birth weight is less than 500 g have a poor prognosis and comfort care may be a more suitable option for these babies (more about extreme prematurity and resuscitation decisions below).

There are many important things to consider when dealing with preterm infants in relation to their immediate, short- and longer term health. Things which need to be done differently immediately after birth for premature infants are outlined below.

Resuscitation at birth for premature babies

As mentioned above, if you're not at a TERTIARY CENTRE consider transferring the baby whilst still *in utero* so the mother can deliver in a location where the baby will receive specialist care from the very beginning.

The basic principles apply in the same way as for term infants but with more by way of intervention needed at each stage as a basic level of care. Recommendations vary depending on the extremity of prematurity.

Key recommendations by gestational age are as follows.

All preterm babies
■ **Use a lower pressure for inflation breaths**. The pressure of inflation breaths delivered should be reduced to 20–25 cm H_2O for preterm babies. However, if their lungs are deficient of surfactant they will be less compliant and higher pressures may be necessary if inflation breaths are not successful initially.

■ **Consider delayed cord clamping**. For preterm babies born in good condition, there is evidence that delayed clamping of the cord for up to 3 min can reduce the incidence of intraventricular haemorrhage and need for blood transfusions but also means that they are more likely to require phototherapy (Rabe et al. 2004).

■ **Put a warm hat on their head**. Premature babies can lose heat even more rapidly than term babies so put a hat on as well as drying and wrapping them.

Preterm babies less than 32 weeks
■ **Consider giving a small amount of oxygen**. These babies may require a 'blend' of oxygen and air in order to achieve the same oxygen saturations as a TERM BABY. However, too much oxygen can be damaging for these babies and saturation levels must be carefully monitored. Oxygen saturations should not exceed the normal levels for preterm infants for any given number of minutes of age and also should not exceed 95%. Start with 30% oxygen and titrate as needed.

Preterm babies less than 28 weeks
■ **Wrap the baby's body in a plastic bag and put on a hat**. These babies are born with much lower stores of brown fat than term babies, meaning that they get cold much more quickly. They also have a much larger surface area to mass ratio than term babies which contributes to them losing heat more quickly and means that they can become dehydrated very rapidly through evaporation. To try to counter these problems, extremely preterm babies are put in a plastic bag, without drying, immediately after delivery. The first time you see this you may find it rather bizarre, they look like a boil-in-a-bag baby with their little head poking out of the top, but it is a very effective way of prev enting heat and water loss. As for term babies, these babies should be kept under an overhead heater whilst you are resuscitating them.

■ **Give surfactant after delivery and maternal steroids in labour**. Premature babies do not have sufficient surfactant in their lungs which can cause problems with respiration. Giving steroids to mothers who are going to deliver a preterm infant can help with this and also administration of surfactant directly into the baby's lungs following delivery has been shown to significantly reduce neonatal morbidity and mortality. Surfactant must be given via an endotracheal tube and therefore this is certainly not something you will be expected to do without senior input.

Extreme prematurity and resuscitation decisions

Your local hospital policy will dictate where these extremes can be pushed to. Generally speaking, any babies born at less than 23 weeks are thought not to be viable and standard practice is to not attempt resuscitation (Wilkinson et al. 2009). Also, standard practice is for babies older than 25 weeks to be resuscitated and treated. The weeks in between are where practice is unclear and there is no real consensus. Specialist units may fairly routinely resuscitate and treat babies as young as 23 weeks. Caring for extremely premature babies is an ethical minefield and can be very upsetting at times. *See Chapter 10 for tips on how to cope with the stress this can put on you.*

One of the big problems is that it is very difficult to predict which babies at the borderline of viability will survive and even more difficult to predict which will survive and be free from significant DISABILITY. Research continues in this area and there have been national studies in the UK to assess survival and long-term morbidity outcomes for extremely premature babies. Whilst survival rates in babies born at 24 weeks' gestation increased significantly between 1995 and 2006, there was no significant change in the survival rates or early major morbidity for those born in the 23rd week (EPICure 2 Perinatal Group 2008). The harsh reality for babies born in the 23rd week is that only 11% survive to be discharged from hospital, of whom two-thirds will have a moderate or severe DISABILITY (Marlow et al. 2005).

Discussions with parents and other healthcare professionals can be complex and compelling arguments may be put forward for opposing decisions. It is extremely important for parents to be informed of all the latest evidence regarding their baby's likelihood of survival and risks of disability in a way which they can understand. For these reasons, it should be a senior doctor having these kinds of discussions with parents but you can learn a huge amount by asking if you can be present. If you have spent significant time caring for a baby then your opinion regarding what is in that baby's

---

Ethical Dilemma

Baby x is born at 23 + 3 gestation by spontaneous vaginal delivery. His mother delivered very soon after arriving at the labour ward and therefore there has been no time to discuss with her and the baby's father regarding resuscitation decisions. The baby appears to be in reasonable condition at birth and you resuscitate as needed and transfer to the neonatal unit (which happens to be a TERTIARY CENTRE).

After the baby has been admitted to the unit, the consultant explains to the parents the implications of being born so prematurely. The parents are keen to do 'whatever is necessary to keep him alive'.

What is in the 'best interests' of this baby? Is it preserving life at all costs? What happens if the parents and healthcare professionals cannot agree regarding this?

---

best interests may also be considered as part of the discussion.

There will probably be guidance at your hospital for procedure after the death of a baby. It may be helpful to refer bereaved parents to the Stillbirth and Neonatal Death Charity website (www.uk-sands.org). Write down the web address or name of the charity for them as they are unlikely to remember it given the situation.

It is important to remember that there is often no 'right answer' in these cases and the guidance available on the subject is largely there to help provide a structure for thinking through difficult cases, not rules on what to do and when. It is important to be aware of key legal issues to be considered in such cases too.

The law in the United Kingdom

Best interests

It is normally considered that the parents of a child will make decisions that are in the 'best interests' of the child and they are granted PARENTAL RESPONSIBILITY. However, there may be occasions when a doctor does not agree that the parents are acting in the child's best interests and can seek permission from the court to overrule their decisions regarding medical treatment. This can be very tricky as defining what is in someone's best interests is a very subjective thing (see section on Useful ethical frameworks and guidance below for some things to think about when considering best interests).

Parental responsibility

Doctors must normally have consent from parents in order provide any treatment for a child or baby. Doctors can only act without parental consent in an emergency or with a court order (which normally only takes a few hours to obtain if urgent). NB: In the UK mothers automatically have PARENTAL RESPONSIBILITY and fathers also have parental responsibility *if* they are married to the mother. If the parents are unmarried then whether or not the father has parental responsibility is complicated – see *the section on consent in Chapter 3 for more details*.

Euthanasia is illegal

Taking direct action with the primary purpose of ending a person's life is illegal regardless of how old they are. From the minute a baby is born, they have the same human rights as any other person. This should not be confused with the *fetus* having legal rights. Until a baby is born, under English law, they have no independent legal status.

Intending relief of distress is normally legal

Motivation is key here. If a doctor gives a patient morphine in order to relieve their pain and suffering (whilst recognising that this may shorten that patient's life) then this is normally legal if the patient is likely to die soon anyway and the dose of morphine is reasonable. The primary intended outcome was pain relief rather than expediting death. This does not mean that death can be a reasonable method of relieving someone's pain – that is euthanasia.

Withdrawing or withholding treatment is the same in the eyes of the law

For example, if you stop a baby's ventilatory support this is viewed as the same as deciding never to start the baby on ventilation. This means that you can withdraw treatment on the same grounds as withholding treatment, e.g. that treatment is futile or that it is in the patient's best interests not to give the treatment.

Some useful ethical frameworks and guidance

What is in a child's best interests? What constitutes a 'good quality of life'? When should withdrawing or withholding of treatment be considered? These are all thorny questions and vary case by case but the following may help you to think them through.

The Royal College of Paediatrics and Child Health has published guidance for when withholding or withdrawing treatment may be considered in children. The 'no chance' and 'no purpose' scenarios are most relevant to neonatology (Ethics Advisory Committee Group 2004).

I Brainstem death – this can only be assessed in older children and must meet certain criteria for diagnosis.

2 Permanent vegetative state – again this one is probably more applicable to older children.

3 'No chance' – despite all treatment, there is no chance of the child surviving and treatment prolongs suffering and the process of dying.

4 'No purpose' – the child may survive if given the necessary interventions but they will be so impaired that their quality of life would be unacceptable.

5 'Unbearable' – the treatment would cause such suffering as to be worse than the disease itself.

The latest version of this guidance from 2004 also contains a small section specifically relating to care of neonates – it can be found on the RCPCH website.

Another very useful resource is a report published by the Nuffield Council on Bioethics in 2006 regarding the ethical issues surrounding care of the neonate. The short guide of this report isn't too long and gives a great overview of the issues to consider. It can be found at www.nuffieldbioethics.org

Intravenous fluids in infants

Some babies admitted to the neonatal unit will need intravenous fluids if they are unable to feed sufficiently to meet their fluid requirements or if it is not safe for them to feed orally.

There is no one standard regime for prescribing fluids for infants as their fluid requirements will vary based on their gestation, weight, how many days old they are and also their environment (for example, the humidity and heat of their incubator). Many units will use something similar to the regime in the table below in order to calculate total fluid requirements for a normal TERM BABY.

Day of life	Total volume of fluid required per day
1	60 mL/kg
2	90 mL/kg
3	120 mL/kg
4 days and older	150 mL/kg

These numbers represent the *total* volume of fluid a baby is likely to need (i.e. the sum of any oral, nasogastric and intravenous fluid). This means that as babies start to increase the amount of oral fluid they can tolerate, their additional intravenous fluid should be reduced accordingly.

The standard fluid of choice for infants is normally 10% dextrose with electrolytes being added to the fluids if needed.

The 'Neonatal Intensive Care' section of the paediatrics.co.uk website has an online calculator to work out a baby's fluid and electrolyte requirements by entering their gestation, weight and date of birth.

Neonatal nurses

Neonatal nurses are highly specialised and skilled people and (as long as you get them on side) they will help you enormously as you are learning how neonatology works. Many are able to take bloods and cannulate so if you play your cards right they may do some of these for you and/or teach you how to do them yourself. If the neonatal nurses like you, it will make your job a *lot* easier. Other than the usual courtesies, here are some specifics which may help.

■ If taking blood or putting in a cannula, use paper towels to stop blood from getting all over the sheets and the baby's clothes

■ Try to leave things (including the baby) as you found them, e.g. baby lying in same position, incubator doors closed, etc.

■ Openly admit when you don't know and ask for their advice.

Useful websites

www.paediatrics.co.uk: has useful information for neonates including an online calculator for working out neonatal fluid and electrolyte requirements.

www.resus.org.uk: for all the latest resuscitation guidance.

http://newborns.stanford.edu/PhotoGallery/General.html: gallery of common abnormalities found on newborn baby checks.

www.uk-sands.org: charity which provides support to bereaved parents of newborns.

www.epicure.ac.uk: website for the large national trials collecting data for very premature babies.

www.nuffieldbioethics.org: contains useful guidance on the ethics surrounding neonatal care.

http://www.nhs.uk/start4life: useful information for parents about health in pregnancy and caring for a newborn baby.

References

Apgar V (1953) A proposal for a new method of evaluation of the newborn infant. *Curr Res Anesth Analg* **32**(4): 260–267.

Cave S, Fertleman C (2007) *Your Baby Week by Week*. Vermilion, London.

EPICure 2 Perinatal Group (2008) Survival and early morbidity of extremely preterm babies in England: changes since 1995. *Arch Dis Child* **93**(Suppl 1): A33–34.

Ethics Advisory Committee Group (2004) *Withholding or Withdrawing Life Sustaining Treatment in Children: A Framework for Practice*. Royal College of Paediatrics and Child Health, London. www.rcpch.ac.uk

Marlow N, Wolke D, Bracewell MA, Samara M for the EPICure Study Group (2005) Neurologic and developmental disability at six years of age after extremely preterm birth. *N Engl J Med* **352**: 9–19.

Nuffield Council on Bioethics (2006) *Critical Care Decisions in Fetal and Neonatal Medicine: Ethical Issues*. Nuffield Council on Bioethics, London.

Rabe H, Reynolds G, Diaz-Rossello J (2004) Early versus delayed umbilical cord clamping in preterm infants. *Cochrane Database Syst Rev* **4**: CD003248.

Wilkinson A, Ahluwalia J, Cole A, et al. (2009) Management of babies born extremely preterm at less than 26 weeks gestation: a framework for clinical practice at the time of birth. *Arch Dis Child Fetal Neonatal Ed* **94**: 2–5.

Chapter 10
LOOKING AFTER YOURSELF

Looking after yourself isn't just crucial for your own health, it's also important for your patients. If you're exhausted, stressed or starving hungry, your clinical judgement will not be as good as normal and you will probably have much less patience when dealing with families.

Some days it can feel like you barely have time to take a breath and rush madly from one thing to the next. In fact, the best thing you can do to increase your efficiency may be to sit down, even for just 10 min, and have something to eat or drink, reorder your thoughts, take a deep breath and start again.

Dealing with upsetting situations

Being a doctor, by its very nature, involves working with people who are unwell and the emotional distress which comes with that. At times paediatrics can involve the most extreme examples of human emotions – for the child, their parents and the staff who care for them. It is important to find ways of dealing with the immediate impact of such situations and also with the chronic stress involved in caring for other people. Prioritising looking after yourself and finding ways to cope is not self-indulgent, it is vital for your long-term success as a doctor.

Short-term coping mechanisms

There will be times when something upsetting happens at work and you need to find a way of getting through the rest of the day. Giving yourself some time to recover before moving on to the next patient can help to ensure that your mind is focused again. Everyone has their own ways of dealing with things but you might find some of the following helpful.

■ **Talk to colleagues**.

– **Formal support**. Many paediatric departments will have a debriefing session following upsetting events (such as child protection cases, prolonged resuscitation or the death of a child) in order for those involved to process what has happened. Some units also run regular meetings for trainees to discuss issues which they have found troubling or upsetting. Normally these are facilitated by someone impartial (such as a

The Hands-on Guide to Practical Paediatrics, First Edition. Rebecca Hewitson and Caroline Fertleman.
© 2014 John Wiley & Sons, Ltd. Published 2014 by John Wiley & Sons, Ltd.
Companion Website: www.wileyhandsonguides.com/paediatrics

CAMHS doctor) or involve trainees only. This can be a useful opportunity to talk openly with your peers and it can be reassuring to find that other people are struggling with the same issues.

– **Informal support**. Finding a few moments to sit and talk with colleagues can help, particularly those who have been involved in whatever has happened. If a child who has been known to members of the team for a long time dies, some people find it helpful to attend the funeral service or to arrange an informal gathering with colleagues away from the hospital to remember the life of that child and share memories and stories about time spent with them.

■ **Be prepared**. One of the hardest things to deal with can be the breaking of bad news to families and your response to their grief. Managing this well can have an enormous impact for these families but also for helping you to cope with the situation. *For advice on breaking bad news see Chapter 3 – Communication with Children and Their Parents.*

■ **Don't be afraid to cry about it**. This is something which doctors are often terrified of doing as they fear being perceived as weak or unprofessional. In fact, families do not perceive this as weakness but as a sign of how much you cared for their child; a survey of bereaved parents found that professionals delivering bad news with genuine empathy for their grief were perceived as much better than those who were 'business-like' (Finlay and Dallimore 1991). Obviously, it is important that your reactions are proportionate and that you maintain composure but

sometimes it is all right to shed a few tears with families who are grieving. Finding a quiet place where you will not be disturbed for 5 min to go and cry on your own can allow you to continue much more effectively with the rest of your shift rather than swallowing back your emotions and ending up dwelling on it all day.

■ **Take a few minutes to be by yourself**. Go for a short walk around the outside of the hospital, go for a cup of tea, sit quietly in the hospital chapel or listen to some music. Whatever it is you choose, give yourself 5 min to take a few deep breaths and feel calmer before getting back to work.

■ **Humour**. Doctors often use humour to help them cope with difficult emotional situations. This can be useful for some people but be aware of your impact on others. Colleagues may assume that you are callous or uncaring if they don't realise that this is your way of coping so be sensitive to this. Similarly, overhearing laughter (even about something entirely unrelated) will feel devastating to families who are grieving.

■ **Sometimes you may not feel anything**. Experiencing no emotional response at all can be even more alarming than feeling upset. There is no 'right' way to respond to a situation and your reaction may differ from that of your colleagues or between different patients and scenarios. This initial detachment may be followed by emotions later on once you have had time to process what has happened. If you find that you are feeling numb and detached from patients and their

> **Box 10.1** Some symptoms of Burnout (Kearney et al. 2009)
>
> ■ Poor decision making and increase in errors
> ■ Perfectionism and an inflexible approach
> ■ Physical and emotional exhaustion that doesn't improve following time off
> ■ Cynical, detached approach to patients
> ■ Irritability and frequent arguments with colleagues
> ■ Apathy and low motivation
> ■ Insomnia and fatigue
> ■ Social withdrawal and isolation

> **Box 10.2** The five stages of grieving
>
> People are thought to go through five different stages when coming to terms with death, whether it be their own or that of someone else (Kübler-Ross 1969). Not everyone will go through all of these stages and not necessarily in this order but being aware of them may be helpful.
>
> ■ **Denial and isolation.** It is normal to rationalise overwhelming emotions and many doctors will focus purely on medical or intellectual things as a way of coping.
>
> ■ **Anger.** This can come out as arguments with colleagues or with your friends and family when you leave work. You may focus on small things which you become furious about, possibly even things related to the way the case was handled.
>
> ■ **Bargaining.** What if we'd done this differently? What if we'd made the diagnosis more quickly?
>
> ■ **Depression.** You may find yourself becoming tearful or more withdrawn than usual.
>
> ■ **Acceptance.**

families quite frequently then this could be a sign of burnout (see Box 10.1 for signs and symptoms of burnout).

■ **Your feelings may change over time**. Your emotional response to an event may alter as time passes. This is a frequent bereavement reaction and sometimes following the death of a patient you have worked with closely, you may experience bereavement in the same way as you would if a friend or family member died. See Box 10.2 for the five stages involved in coming to terms with death.

Long-term coping mechanisms

Stress is the immediate reaction to a difficult situation, but burnout happens after this has continued for a long time. Everyone has days that leave them feeling stressed or tired but burnout is when, even after time off between shifts, you don't recover. Burnout is actually a recognised and defined problem but one which is rarely talked about. Symptoms of prolonged stress and burnout are very common amongst doctors and this has implications for the quality of patient care, not just the quality of those doctors' lives (Firth-Cozens 2003). *See Box 10.1 for symptoms of burnout.*

Recognising symptoms of stress in yourself and others is one thing, but how do you go about alleviating it? Some of the protective factors against burnout are to do with the environment in which you work but there are also ways in which you can control your own behaviours. There is evidence from randomised trials to suggest that practising mindful meditation and reflective writing can be helpful in preventing burnout (Kearney et al. 2009); other interventions such as work-based programmes are still being studied. Many of the other things listed below have little evidence base in reference specifically to doctors but are part of the widespread advice we give to patients about handling stress so perhaps we ought to pay more heed to ourselves.

■ **Meditation**. Time and time again when talking to doctors who don't seem stressed, despite busy schedules and demanding jobs, I find that they practise meditation. There is also some evidence to suggest that this can make doctors more self-aware and better at listening to their patients (Beckman et al. 2012). In fact, several medical schools have even incorporated mindfulness into their curriculum (Hutchinson and Dobkin 2009).

■ **Reflective writing**. Keeping a reflective log is often thought of as another hurdle to jump in a long list of tedious work-based assessments, but if you use it well it can be enormously helpful. Using a structured way of reflecting (see *Box 10.3*), can help you work through what happened, and why, and to come up with constructive solutions for what you will change if you come across a similar situation in future. This is a powerful way of improving your practice and can help you to take something positive away from a bad situation and move on rather than dwelling on what happened. Reflective writing forms a key part of the GMC revalidation process, which all doctors must now undergo every 5 years. It is all right (and only human) to make mistakes but the important thing is that you can show that you are capable of reflecting on what happened in order to learn from it and improve your practice. Sometimes, writing a formal reflective piece, which others may read, may not be appropriate immediately, but you may find it helpful to write in a diary. This can allow you to write freely and fully acknowledge your emotional response to the situation. You may find that it is later useful to complete a formal reflection on the same subject once you have had time to distance yourself from your immediate emotional responses.

Box 10.3 Some examples of structure frameworks for reflecting

The Gibbs framework for reflective practice (Gibbs 1988)

1 **Describe** – What happened? Who was there? Don't forget to remove any patient identifiable information.

2 **Self-awareness** – What were you thinking? What were you feeling?

3 **Evaluation** – What was good about the experience? What was bad?

4 **Analysis** – What do you think other people would have done? What evidence is there for what should happen or how to avoid similar situations?

5 **Conclusions** – Both general and specific about what happened and why. What could you have done differently?

6 **Action plan** – What will you do differently next time? Is there anything you need to do to ensure that this will happen?

Or if you find the Gibbs framework too lengthy, an easy one to remember is the What? reflection model which asks three questions (Borton 1970, Gibbs 1988).

1 **What?** – Describe what happened. What was good or bad about it?

2 **So what?** – Why is it important? What have you learnt?

3 **Now what?** – What are you going to do now? How will you act differently in future?

Alternatively, you can write it formally but keep the page locked (i.e. with a password) and then you might want to unlock it later on or share it only with one other person.

■ **Hobbies**. Remember how when you were applying for medical school you had a personal statement crammed full of all the extracurricular things you did? Many of those previous hobbies may seem like a distant memory now but they are more important than ever once you start working. The whole point of selecting medical students who have a wide range of interests is so that once they are doctors, they will have constructive ways

of relaxing that don't always involve getting drunk! Make time for these previous hobbies or try something totally new and different. Whatever it is, make sure that you prioritise time for enjoying yourself. At times, it may feel that all you do is work, eat and sleep but even having one thing to look forward to each week or each fortnight can be enough to keep you going through the worst.

■ **Exercise**. Find some form of physical activity that you enjoy, or at the very least work it into your daily routine so that it becomes habit (taking the stairs instead of the lift, cycling to work). It shouldn't become another chore or it defeats the point; find what it is that you enjoy and make time for it. Taking exercise to relieve stress is something we advise our patients to do; the key is finding a way to take your own advice.

■ **Friends and family**. Talking things over with someone you care about can help enormously as can having someone around to cheer you up and distract you. Do your best to keep in touch with friends and family even when you're working a busy rota. It can sometimes feel like you're too exhausted to see anyone at all, but this can be the very time that you most need to make the effort to get out and see people. Putting in a small amount of effort to go and meet up with someone you care about can leave you feeling far more energised than an extra hour in bed.

■ **Coaching and mentoring**. Coaching sessions can be a very useful way of working through specific challenges by helping you to find answers for yourself. There are coaching and mentoring schemes available in some deaneries, often provided by a medical professional trained in coaching but from a different specialty (so that they will never be someone to whom you answer for clinical work). Look at the Support4Doctors website (www.support4doctors.org) under 'Search for organisations that can help' for a list of available coaching and mentoring services. Alternatively, if there is not one available in your area you could consider paying for private coaching sessions or try to set up a scheme at your deanery. The London Deanery coaching and mentoring scheme is well established and would be a good place to start for advice about setting up your own (http://mentoring.londondeanery.ac.uk).

Bullying and harassment

Stressful and upsetting situations at work are not just confined to our interactions with patients; relationships with colleagues can sometimes be difficult to manage too. Getting on badly with some of your colleagues or being around colleagues who don't get on with one another can be very stressful. Witnessing or being subject to bullying is also very distressing. Most trusts will have their own antibullying or equality and diversity guidelines. The BMA also has a useful guide on its website. Some key points to consider if you are witnessing or experiencing bullying include the following.

■ Talk to a supervisor or senior colleague whom you trust to raise your concerns.

■ Consult your trust's antibullying policy.

■ Keep a diary of incidents to refer back to.

■ Consider contacting the human resources department at your hospital for advice.

■ Check your deanery or local education trust board website – there may be local advice and support available.

■ If you are a student, raise the issue with your medical school who should have a dedicated member of staff who deals with pastoral issues.

Practising paediatrics when you have your own children

Fulfilling dual roles of being a doctor and a parent can be very challenging at times. Working out the practicalities of childcare and shift work can be a tricky balancing act and combining the two roles can sometimes involve situations which trigger strong emotions. But being a parent also has the potential to make you a better doctor and many families will be heartened by paediatricians who have their own children.

Below are some of the challenges doctors who are parents sometimes face, along with possible solutions and how these challenges can help you develop skills which make you a better doctor.

Emotional impact

■ **The challenge.** Sometimes the most upsetting situations can be those involving people who remind us of our own family members. This can be particularly hard if you are looking after a sick child who is a similar age to your own. Witnessing the grief of parents or the suffering of a child can be much more painful for some people once they have children of their own.

■ **How this can be a strength.** Having children of your own can deepen your understanding of what families and parents are going through. Knowing first hand some of the challenges parents face can make it easier to anticipate their questions and properly address their concerns. This certainly does not mean that your experiences of parenting will be the same as everyone else's but it will give you a useful starting point. Having your own children can also give you a much better feel for the range of what is normal.

■ **Potential solutions.** You may find it helpful to talk to colleagues who have children of their own. This doesn't just have to be other doctors; it can be useful to talk to nursing colleagues and other members of the multidisciplinary team as well.

Not enough hours in the day

■ **The challenge.** Being a parent and being a doctor are both very time-consuming roles and parents can end up feeling guilty about having to compromise either on time with their children or time spent at work. Childcare arrangements can sometimes be very restrictive, meaning that you have to leave work at a fixed time, which can occasionally cause resentment from colleagues.

■ **How this can be a strength.** These added time pressures can help you to develop excellent time management skills and you may find that you become much more efficient at work as a result. Splitting your time between childcare and work also adds variety to your life and may allow you to approach both with a greater enthusiasm than if you were solely doing one or the other.

■ **Potential solutions.** Investing in decent childcare can put your mind at

Top Tip

Traditionally paternity leave has only been 2 weeks long, compared to maternity leave of up to 52 weeks. However, it is currently possible to apply for additional paternity leave in some cases and there are big changes planned in the UK. If it is passed through Parliament, the Children and Families Bill will put in place 'parental leave' instead of the traditional maternity and paternity leave. This would mean that (after the compulsory 2 weeks of maternity leave following delivery) parents are free to split the remainder of the parental leave as they choose. This gives much more flexibility, can free up time for both parents to spend with their new baby and can minimise the impact on both careers.

rest and help with some of the time restraints. If you are expecting a baby, look into this before they are born as there are often waiting lists for good childcare facilities. For advice on how to find good childcare services, see the less than full-time training page on the RCPCH website and for information on the financial support available for childcare go to www.gov.uk. Sometimes it may be difficult to leave on time, particularly if your colleagues are not very sympathetic, but don't be afraid to be assertive. If you need to pick your child up from childcare then you do need to go so don't feel guilty about it. If you find that colleagues are becoming resentful,

you can offer to help them out in other ways – try to swap shifts if you can or offer to take on some of the boring jobs that day if you know you will need to leave early. You may wish to train less than full time for a while in order to free up more time to spend with your children. *For more information on less than full-time training see Chapter 11 – Developing Your Career.*

Feeling isolated

■ **The challenge**. Although graduate entry medicine is increasingly common, you will probably still find that most of your peers do not yet have children. This may make you feel quite isolated as your lives outside work may be very different and you may occasionally miss out on socialising with colleagues because of childcare responsibilities.

■ **How this can be a strength**. By having children earlier on in your career, you will be free to take on more responsibilities later on once they are older and you are working at a more senior level. Lots of your colleagues may not have children until they are registrars or consultants and therefore will not want to take on additional work during this time. If by this stage your children are older and you have more free time, you can make the most of the additional opportunities which result.

■ **Potential solutions**. Finding colleagues who are also parents can give you someone to talk to and the chance to learn from their experiences and share some of the challenges. Colleagues whose children are older than yours can be useful mentors and can prove that it is possible to survive even the toughest bits. If there is no-one in your department whom you feel comfortable talking to, you can find contacts and support through other organisations such as the Medical Women's Federation (www.medicalwomensfederation.org.uk) or general parenting support groups such as Family Lives (http://familylives.org.uk).

Nobody's perfect: dealing with mistakes

Dealing with situations where we've done something wrong is really unpleasant as there is a combined fear of having caused harm to a patient and of being punished or humiliated by your seniors or the GMC.

Owning up to your mistakes is essential, even if you dread the conversation with patients, their relatives and your colleagues. Trying to cover up a mistake will bring your honesty and integrity into question which can have much graver implications from a disciplinary point of view than the mistake itself.

Human nature means that we all make mistakes sometimes and the important thing is learning how to deal with them when they happen and how to prevent the same mistake from happening again.

Key things to do when you realise you've made a mistake include the following.

■ **Apologise**. Swallow your pride and go to the patient and their relatives and say that you are sorry. However, saying things like 'I'm sorry but…' or 'I'm sorry that you feel that way' is *not* an apology.

■ **Sort out any immediate safety concerns**. As soon as you realise your mistake, take any medical action needed to prevent further harm to the patient.

■ **Involve senior colleagues**. It is best to involve your senior colleagues at the earliest opportunity. This will allow them to help you with any medical action which needs to be taken and with discussions with the family (and other members of the team if necessary) about what happened.

■ **Answer questions**. Do your best to answer any questions the patient and their relatives have about what happened, why and what will be done to put any issues right. It may be helpful to do this with one of your senior colleagues present to answer any difficult questions you are unsure about.

■ **Fill in an incident form**. This can seem tedious but is actually very important and not done anywhere near frequently enough. To you, it might seem trivial but recording your error allows hospital management to look at trends across the entire organisation. It may be that lots of people are making the same mistake and that it is the processes and systems involved which need to be changed. It can be helpful to tell the family that you plan to do this in order to prevent similar incidents from happening in the future.

■ **Reflect on what happened**. Writing a structured reflection about what happened and why can help you to work out how you need to alter your practice and what specific things you will do differently next time in order to avoid making similar mistakes in the future. *See Box 10.3 for some structured frameworks for reflection.*

■ **Call your defence union**. If you're really worried you can discuss with your defence union to take its advice about difficult cases. However, you don't need to wait until a crisis happens to call your defence union; it can offer advice and support on many relatively minor or routine things too. For example, it has a legal team who can read through any formal statements or reports you have to make (for example, in child protection cases).

Avoiding making mistakes

Being able to deal with mistakes when they happen is important but there are also ways to reduce the risk of them happening in the first place. Preventing mistakes is about personal responsibility but also about creating systems which minimise the possibility of human error resulting in harm to a patient. *For more information about how you can improve the environment in which you work and make things safer for patients, see Chapter 11 – Developing Your Career.*

Although it is clear that the environment in which we work is important, there are also things which we can do as individuals to reduce the risk of making mistakes. Having an awareness of some common themes in cases of medical error may help you to avoid

these pitfalls yourself. So what things frequently go wrong and what can you do to avoid them?

Pitfall 1: Communication

The most common theme in all major medical errors is that poor communication between different members of the team was a major factor in allowing the error to occur. Small errors in the information communicated between different members of the team can culminate in one large error being made with huge consequences for the patient. Communicating well isn't just about getting on well and being nice to members of your team (although that certainly helps); it is about making sure that everyone understands what is happening and that important messages get through to the relevant people.

What can you do about it?

■ **Listen properly** to what someone is telling you. Don't carry on with what you are doing and not pay proper attention as this can mean that you miss important information. Stop what you are doing and actually look at the person talking to you. This is not just the polite thing to do but it also means that you can pick up on non-verbal cues which might be telling you so much more than simply the words they are saying.

■ **Use communication tools**. Simple ways of communicating information effectively can improve the efficiency of things like handover as well as improving safety. *See Box 10.4 for examples of two commonly used communication tools.*

Box 10.4 Two commonly used communication tools

The **Paediatric Early Warning Score (PEWS)** is a useful way of getting a quick snapshot idea of how well or unwell a child is. It is calculated using the child's observations, with abnormal observations being allocated a particular score. If all observations are within normal range then the child will have a PEWS score of 0. The higher the PEWS score, the more unwell the child. The maximum score is 6.

SBAR is very useful for concise communication of information. SBAR stands for Situation, Background, Assessment and Recommendations. For more about how to use SBAR, including teaching resources and videos of a handover using SBAR, go to the NHS Institute for Innovation and Improvement website (www.institute.nhs.uk/SBAR). Here is a brief description of how to use it at handover with an example.

■ **Situation** – if you were writing a newspaper article, this would be the headline. It is one sentence which sums up the key points, e.g. 'Ben is a 10-year-old boy who was admitted overnight with a painful sickle cell crisis. He is currently stable with a PEWS score of 1 and is on patient-controlled analgesia and IV fluids'.

■ **Background** – presenting complaint and brief history. Relevant past medical history. What was the child like when they first presented? For example, 'Ben presented with severe left leg pain which feels the same as his normal sickle cell pain. His crisis may have been triggered by going to the ice-rink yesterday. He has had five previous admissions with painful crises, the latest one was in February last year following a viral illness'.

■ **Assessment** – how is the child now? What is their PEWS score? What are their relevant examination findings and investigation results? 'Ben's initial pain score at presentation was 8 out of 10 and he was given a 50 microgram/kg dose of intravenous morphine. He is now on a patient-controlled analgesia pump which he is currently using every 1–2 h and reports that his pain score is currently 6. His PEWS score is currently 1, for a tachycardia of 120. On examination he has no signs of respiratory distress and his chest sounds clear. His haemoglobin is 7.6 which is normal for him (his haemoglobin is usually between 6 and 8.5), with an appropriately raised reticulocyte count of 2.5% (again this is normal range for him).'

■ **Recommendations** – what treatment is ongoing? What needs to happen to this treatment? Any specialist reviews needed? Any results need chasing? 'I recommend continued monitoring of fluid balance and considering stopping his intravenous fluids today if he is drinking sufficiently. He will need to have his pain medication reviewed today with a view to converting him to oral analgesia if tolerated. He will need to be seen by the specialist sickle cell nurse today too. There are no pending results to be chased.'

■ **Use good-quality written communication**. Whether this be keeping the patient list up to date, recording accurately in the medical notes or writing complete discharge summaries, the quality of written communication is really important. This is crucial for transfer of information between day-time and night-time teams, between different hospitals and to the child's GP. Poor communication between different teams is not only a source of extreme frustration for that child's family but leaves all professionals very vulnerable to making errors. Writing good-quality discharge and transfer letters can help enormously with this. For particularly complex cases, sending a photocopy of the child's most recent medication chart, medical notes and blood results may help the receiving hospital team to understand exactly what has been done already and why.

■ **Raise your concerns**. Sometimes when medical errors are investigated, junior members of the team will say that they realised at the time that something was not right or that they could see what needed to be done but lacked the courage to say so. It is crucial to speak up if you think that one of your senior colleagues has got something wrong as they are just as vulnerable to making errors as everyone else and will probably be grateful for your support. If you are trying to tell someone something important, make sure that they have definitely heard you and have processed what you are telling them. You can do this politely but don't be afraid to be assertive if you feel that

they have not properly listened to important information.

Pitfall 2: Being distracted at a critical moment

Avoiding making mistakes requires concentration and if you are not fully focused on a task because of a distraction or you are interrupted part way through doing something, this can increase your risk of making a mistake.

What can you do about it?

■ **Be considerate of other team members**. You may have noticed that nurses doing a drug round now often wear a red bib which says 'Do not disturb' on it or that nurses are particularly annoyed if you interrupt them when there are two of them in the drug room checking a medication dose. This is because the measuring out and checking of medication doses are two critical points for patient safety and it can be really dangerous if you distract them at these times and cause them to make a mistake. It can be frustrating at times if you need to ask about something and the nurse you need is busy, but make a point of not interrupting unless it is a real emergency. Having a message board or space on a white board with patient names to inform nurses of any changes you have made to the treatment plan is a useful way of communicating key information without interrupting.

■ **Establish clear rules**. Just as many departments have worked out ways for nursing staff to carry out drug rounds safely, it might be useful to come up with ways for you to avoid distractions and interruptions. An obvious example is when you are prescribing. This can apply to discharge medications as well as to prescribing when on the ward round. Agreeing with colleagues that the person prescribing shouldn't be interrupted adds a safety mechanism into your routine.

■ **Don't distract yourself**. It can be tempting when you're really busy to try to multi-task to save time. This is fine for some things but for safety-critical things like prescribing, it is a really bad idea as it leaves you vulnerable to making mistakes. You can also be distracted in the middle of something important if your phone starts ringing – leave it somewhere safe or keep it in silent mode if you have to carry it with you.

Pitfall 3: Failure to follow protocol

Many hospitals will have protocols to follow for emergency care or certain treatments. Failing to follow an established protocol is dangerous and indefensible unless you have a really good reason (for which you may well need senior agreement). The problem can sometimes be remembering that the protocol exists and what it is in times of stress or not knowing about it in the first place.

What can you do about it?
■ **Read in advance**. In an emergency situation it is unlikely that you will have time to check whether or not a protocol exists for management of that condition. Making yourself aware of some

of them (for example, how to manage anaphylaxis or a choking child) by attending Advanced Life Support courses or checking the hospital or national guidelines can allow you to respond appropriately when an emergency happens.

■ **Familiarise yourself with your environment**. Many emergency departments will have key protocols stuck to the wall of each cubicle as a flowchart or available on the CRASH TROLLEY. Similarly, many units will have a copy of the neonatal life support algorithm on the RESUSCITAIRE. Knowing where these are and which scenarios they cover will allow you to check quickly in an emergency.

■ **Ask the patient or their parents**. For some diagnoses patients will have a personalised plan for their care. For example, all paediatric oncology patients will receive investigation, diagnosis and treatment based on agreed national protocols. This lays out all the steps involved in their care and each child will have a personalised plan.

Pitfall 4: Acting beyond your competence

This one doesn't really need much explanation but sadly does still happen on occasion. Never be tempted to act outside of what you are competent to do. If you are unsure about something then ask for help, even if it hurts your pride to do so. It is far better to feel embarrassed at owning up that you don't know how to do something than to risk harming a child.

Organisation

Like it or not, being a junior doctor involves a large administrative burden and means you need to have pretty good organisational skills if you are ever going to leave the hospital on time. This comes quite naturally to some people whilst for others it can be more of a steep learning curve. Regardless of which of these you are, working on your organisational and time management skills can massively reduce the stress of working as a junior doctor. Here are some suggestions you may find helpful in organising and staying on top of your workload.

■ **Write everything down**. This might seem totally obvious but it's very easy to think that you'll remember one small job but get distracted (by a bleep or an emergency) before completing it. Keeping a list of all the jobs you have to do can also allow you to easily see what needs to be done and prioritise.

■ **Prioritise**. Even if you've written everything down, it can be difficult to know where to start! One helpful approach can be simply picking the three most urgent jobs and then labelling them one to three. Do those jobs and then plan the next three once these are done. Using this trick can help reduce your stress levels on hectic days as it helps you to remain focused and avoid becoming overwhelmed by the list as a whole.

■ **Learn from your colleagues**. Pay attention to things that your colleagues do to make their work more efficient. They might be particularly good at keyboard shortcuts, have a clipboard to keep everything they need together, or colour-code their jobs with a multi-colour biro. Some of these are pretty naff but they might mean that you can have a social life because you get everything done on time.

■ **Delegate**. This doesn't mean dumping jobs on to other people, it's about being clear about who is responsible for which job and allocating tasks appropriately. It can be helpful to sit down as a team after the ward round and work out who will do which jobs and write their initials next to each on your own lists or a centrally held one (for example, in the doctors' office). This avoids duplication of work or, worse, some jobs being forgotten completely. It also makes it easier to chase up certain things if you know who is responsible for what.

■ **Anticipate**. Dealing with things before they become an issue can save you a lot of time in the long run. For example, preparing discharge medications at the last minute can end up taking a lot longer because you make mistakes, which the pharmacist then needs to clarify with you and then you have to alter.

■ **Become good at using computers**. A huge chunk of work done by junior doctors involves paperwork and virtually all of this is now done on computers. Most NHS trusts will have about four or five different programmes that you need to use for ordering bloods, checking results, writing discharge summaries, etc. Given that these programmes often differ between trusts too, you will probably find that you have to learn how to use several different programmes each time you start at a new hospital. Once you've learnt the basics, ask a Foundation Year 1 doctor for more tips. Given that FY1 doctors handle the majority of the hospital's administrative burden, they will probably be able to tell you how to avoid annoying glitches and make life faster when using the hospital systems. If you *are* an FY1 doctor, then ask the FY1 who is leaving the job when you first start.

■ **Make use of other technology**. Many people now have smart phones and there are lots of different applications (apps) available which can help make your working life much quicker. For example, rather than spending a long time searching for a paper copy of the BNFc, you can now download it as an app for your phone and this text-book is also available electronically so that you don't have to carry the paper copy with you. There are also apps available with the latest guidelines from the Scottish Intercollegiate Guidelines Network (SIGN) and the National Institute for Health and Clinical Excellence (NICE). *Make sure that you only use apps from trusted sources if you are using them to inform your medical decisions.*

■ **Change the system**. If the current processes used at your hospital are time consuming and inefficient then why not try to think of something better yourself? This will save time not only for you but also for your colleagues who go after you. *For more information about service improvement projects see Chapter 11 – Developing Your Career.*

Night shifts

Some people don't find it too bad switching their body clock to work night shifts, others really struggle. Working night shifts is tiring but many people find that they are a welcome opportunity to see their children in the afternoons or enjoy the reduced administrative burden overnight. Remember to take some food with you for 'lunch' and plenty of water to drink. You may not feel like eating as much as usual but eating something will help keep your energy levels up.

Getting some good sleep in the day time between your shifts can be difficult but makes a world of difference to how well you are able to function on your shifts. Here are some top tips on how to make sure you get some restful sleep.

■ **Black out blinds in your bedroom or an eye mask** – this can work wonders for making sure that you get some decent sleep.

■ **Ear plugs** – there is usually a lot more noise going on during the day, regardless of where you live, so ear plugs can help stop you from being disturbed.

■ **Turn your phone off** – don't get woken up by unwanted text messages or phone calls. If you're concerned that people may want to contact you in an emergency then you can always download apps which allow you to program your phone to be silent for all phone calls apart from certain specified numbers, which will get through. Don't forget to tell the people on your list of numbers

👍 Top Tip

Try to use public transport to get to and from work rather than driving if possible. If you have to drive to work, consider booking a room in the hospital for the duration of your night shifts. This can seem a depressing prospect but actually, downloading lots of films to watch whilst you're there means it can be quite enjoyable. It is really dangerous driving when tired and it is far better to stay at the hospital than risk killing yourself or others on the roads.

that you're working night shifts so that they don't disturb you unnecessarily.

■ **Eat something before you go to bed** – you'll wake up feeling hungry unless you have something to eat before trying to get to sleep.

■ **Go to bed as soon as possible after finishing your shift** – it can be difficult to sleep late into the afternoon so try to avoid getting distracted into doing things when you get home. Have something to eat and then head straight to bed. Everything else can wait until you wake up in the afternoon.

Useful websites

Doctors Support Network: www.dsn.org.uk. This is a fully confidential self-help group for doctors and medical students with mental health concerns (including stress and burnout). There are many links on the website to other related organisations.

Sick Doctors Trust: www.sick-doctors-trust. co.uk. This is a fully confidential organisation which offers support to doctors and medical students who have any degree of dependence on drugs or alcohol. There is a 24-helpline (0370 444 5163).

Support 4 Doctors: www.support4doctors. org. Lots of information and advice on many things from managing stress and physical health to financial and careers advice.

NHS Institute for Innovation and Improvement: http://www.institute.nhs.uk/safer-care. This website contains lots of useful learning resources on patient care including more about the paediatric early warning score and SBAR communication tool.

BMA: www.bma.org.uk. Useful information on careers, practical support and doctors' well-being.

References

Beckman H, Wendland M, Mooney C, et al. (2012) The impact of a program in mindful communication on primary care physicians. *Academic Med* **87**(6): 815–819.

Borton T (1970) *Reach, Touch and Teach*. Hutchinson, London.

Finlay I, Dallimore D (1991) Your child is dead. *BMJ* **302**: 1524–1525.

Firth-Cozens J (2003) Doctors, their wellbeing, and their stress. *BMJ* **326**: 670.

Gibbs G (1988) *Learning by Doing: A Guide to Teaching and Learning Methods*. Further Education Unit, Oxford Polytechnic, Oxford.

Hutchinson H, Dobkin P (2009) Mindful medical practice: just another fad? *Can Fam Physician* **55**(8): 778–779.

Kearney M, Weininger R, Vachon M, Harrison R, Firth-Cozens J (2009) Self-care for physicians caring for patients at the end of life. *JAMA* **301**(11): 1155.

Kübler-Ross E (1969) *On Death and Dying*. Macmillan, New York.

Chapter 11
DEVELOPING YOUR CAREER

Being a doctor involves so much more than just your day-to-day clinical work. It is a continuous process of learning and assessment with a responsibility to ensure that you are providing the best possible care for your patients. There are many challenges (such as passing exams and work-based assessments) but also lots of opportunities to get involved in additional meaningful and rewarding activities such as teaching, working abroad, research and improving the quality of care for patients. This chapter covers the basics and also some information on how to get the most from your career.

Specialist training structure for paediatrics

In the UK, paediatrics is currently a 'run-through' training programme. This means that you apply for the entire training programme needed in order to qualify to work as a consultant in paediatrics. For most doctors this training lasts 8 years but can be longer if you decide to subspecialise, take time 'out of programme' or work part time.

Run-through training means that, as long as you perform well enough, you are guaranteed a post in the same area for the whole of your specialist training. This provides a lot more security and stability than in other specialties where you have to reapply for positions at various different points, but it does mean having to commit to living in the same place for many years. It is possible to transfer to a different area during your specialist training but there are strict national criteria for this which

 Top Tip

The UK was previously divided into 'deaneries' responsible for overseeing the training of doctors working in that geographical area. As a result of the recent NHS reforms (Health and Social Care Act 2012), deaneries have been replaced by Local Education and Training Boards (LETB). Whilst the LETBs will have the same responsibilities as deaneries, the geographical areas that they cover will have changed in some cases so make sure that you have the latest information before applying.

The Hands-on Guide to Practical Paediatrics, First Edition. Rebecca Hewitson and Caroline Fertleman.
© 2014 John Wiley & Sons, Ltd. Published 2014 by John Wiley & Sons, Ltd.
Companion Website: www.wileyhandsonguides.com/paediatrics

apply to all specialties and it is by no means guaranteed that you will be able to move part way through your training. This means that it is important to think carefully when choosing which area to apply to.

Things to consider when choosing a deanery (or LETB) include the following.

■ **Specialist units**. If you are thinking of subspecialising within paediatrics then it is worth considering which deaneries contain hospitals which provide that particular service. Subspecialty training is applied for through a competitive national application process which takes place at level 3 in the training programme (*see Box 11.1 for the structure of paediatrics training in the UK*). In order to increase your chances of success, it is useful to get some experience in your chosen subspecialty during your earlier training years. This will only be possible if you apply to a deanery where there is a unit which provides these services, some of which will only take place at tertiary referral centres.

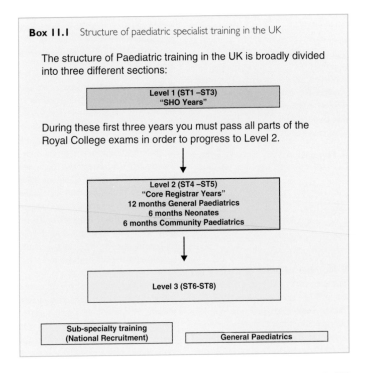

Box 11.1 Structure of paediatric specialist training in the UK

The structure of Paediatric training in the UK is broadly divided into three different sections:

> **Level 1 (ST1 –ST3)**
> **"SHO Years"**

During these first three years you must pass all parts of the Royal College exams in order to progress to Level 2.

> **Level 2 (ST4 –ST5)**
> **"Core Registrar Years"**
> **12 months General Paediatrics**
> **6 months Neonates**
> **6 months Community Paediatrics**

> **Level 3 (ST6-ST8)**

> **Sub-specialty training**
> **(National Recruitment)**

> **General Paediatrics**

■ **Trainee satisfaction**. It is possible to look back at the results of previous national trainee surveys on the GMC website (www.gmc-uk.org/education/surveys), to find out what current paediatric trainees think about different aspects of their training in that deanery. You can look at feedback from trainees about many aspects of working in that deanery such as workload, level of senior support and quality of teaching.

■ **Personal reasons**. Where do you actually want to be living for the next 8 years of your life? Your personal life can change enormously within the space of 8 years so try to think through the possibilities of what might be happening and what might be important to you then as well as now. This is obviously very difficult to predict but talking things through with important people in your life can help you to work out some of what matters to you (and them) now and your collective best guesses for what you might want in the future.

■ **Population**. Who is the population you will be serving? Affluence, ethnic and cultural diversity vary widely between different areas of the UK. Different populations have different disease sets and bring with them their own unique challenges in terms of providing their healthcare.

■ **Number of other trainees**. If you have applied to a deanery where there are only a handful of new paediatric training posts each year, you will very quickly get to know everyone. For some people this is a welcome prospect whilst for others it may feel too claustrophobic.

Information can be found on the RCPCH website about the number of training posts advertised over the past few years in each region and the number of people who applied (http://www.rcpch.ac.uk).

■ **Think really long term**. Although your training years are really important as an experience in themselves, you also need to consider that you will spend the majority of your career as a consultant. Think about what you might like to be doing once you're a consultant and how different training schemes in different regions might help you to get there. It might also be worth considering the number of available consultant posts in the area of your choice and how many trainees from that area are able to find consultant jobs in the same region.

■ **Extra opportunities**. What else does that deanery offer in addition to the normal training? Are there lots of opportunities to become involved in teaching, for example through out-of-programme fellowship schemes? Does the deanery focus on involving their trainees in research? Does it have established leadership and innovation schemes? Each will have a slightly different focus and working out which fits best with your personality and your long-term plans is important. Visit the websites for the different deaneries, talk to people who already work there if possible and attend conferences or careers events at the deaneries you are thinking of applying to. These sorts of things can give you vital clues about the values and aspirations of a particular region and which appeals to you most.

Once you have been accepted onto a paediatric training programme, you become a specialist trainee (ST) and must register as a junior member of the Royal College of Paediatrics and Child Health (which is responsible for overseeing all paediatric training in the UK and ensuring it is of high quality). *See Box 11.1 for an overview of the structure of paediatric training in the UK.*

Opportunities for research

Academic training programme

It is possible to pursue an academic route alongside your specialist training. This pathway is offered by academic clinical fellowship posts or (at a more senior level) academic clinical lectureships, which provide you with the opportunity to split your time between academic and clinical work. You may be able to apply at any level between ST1 and ST4 for an academic clinical fellowship, depending on posts available, and you do not have to have completed an academic foundation programme in order to apply (although this may help). The aim of your academic clinical fellowship is to gain research experience, skills and training, and to secure funding for completion of a higher degree, usually a PhD.

After completion of an academic clinical fellowship, it is expected that many people will go on to complete PhDs and apply for academic clinical lectureships with a view to becoming a consultant with joint academic and clinical responsibilities after they have finished their specialist training. However, it is possible to decide after completion of an academic clinical fellowship that you wish to return to the clinical training pathway instead.

A detailed guide full of valuable practical information about academic training (and written by trainees who have completed academic training themselves) is available on the RCPCH website (RCPCH 2013) (www.rcpch.ac.uk).

For more information about academic clinical fellowships you can also visit the website for the National Institute for Health Research Trainees Co-ordinating Centre (www.nihrtcc.nhs.uk) and also look at the websites for the deaneries to which you are thinking of applying. There is more about the academic medicine pathway available on the medical careers website at www.medicalcareers.nhs.uk.

Out-of-programme research (OOPR)

It is worth noting that you do not have to be an academic clinic fellow in order to conduct research and this can be done as time out of programme instead if you pursue the conventional training programme. *For more information see the Out of Programme section under 'CV building for specialist trainees' above.*

Completing research projects alongside regular training

Taking part in research is useful and important for all trainees as it can give you a greater understanding of how to interpret literature and trial data in order to take a more evidence-based approach to patient management. Smaller projects can certainly be done alongside your regular clinical training if you are dedicated. Approach consultants in your department (or those who conduct research in an area that interests you) to see if they have any research projects you can get involved with.

College exams

In order to become a member of the Royal College of Paediatrics and Child Health (MRCPCH), you must pass several exams. You must pass all the separate parts of the MRCPCH or 'MEMBERSHIP' exams in order to progress to working as a registrar (which starts in ST4 year; see Box 11.1). This can sometimes cause problems as the average time taken by candidates to pass all parts of the MRCPCH is currently 3.5 years but there are only 3 years of specialist training before you are expected to progress to registrar level. This means that some trainees have to delay their progression to working as a registrar whilst attempting to pass the necessary exams. For this reason, amongst others, many people decide to sit some parts of the exam whilst they are a Foundation trainee (more about this below).

The names of the exams and the order in which they can be attempted have recently changed (although the purpose and content of the exams remain more or less the same). It is now possible to sit the written exams in any order you choose (and even sit them all at the same time if you want to), but all written papers must be passed before you can sit the clinical exam.

There are four parts to the MRCPCH: three written papers and one clinical exam.

Written papers

■ **Foundation of Practice (formerly Part 1a)**. This exam consists of one written paper with extended matching, best of five and true or false questions. It aims to test your basic clinical knowledge of paediatrics. Completing a short placement working in paediatrics (even as a Foundation trainee) can be helpful for passing this exam but is by no means essential for success.

■ **Scientific Knowledge and Theory of Practice (formerly Part 1b)**. This exam consists of one written paper with extended matching, best of five and true or false questions. It aims to test your understanding of the science which underpins paediatrics. People often find this the most difficult and historically it has the lowest pass rate of all the written papers. Make sure that you prepare thoroughly for this exam and do plenty of practice questions and background reading.

■ **Applied Knowledge in Practice (Clinical Decision and Management) (formerly Part 2 written)**. This exam is made up of two separate papers, both of which are taken on the same day. These papers focuses primarily on clinical scenarios and your ability to make the correct diagnosis based on a description of history and examination findings, to correctly interpret investigations and to select an appropriate management plan and involvement of colleagues. This exam requires you to have experience working in paediatrics in order to have sufficient clinical knowledge to pass.

Clinical exam

The clinical exam follows an OSCE-style format which you may be familiar with from medical school. You move between different stations all designed to test an aspect of your clinical knowledge and skills.

For more detailed information about the different aspects of the MRCPCH exams, the syllabus and practice papers, visit the Royal College website (www.rcpch.ac.uk). A 'guide for newcomers' can be downloaded from the website with lots of information about each of the exams.

Things to consider when thinking about exams include the following.

■ **Sitting a written paper as a Foundation trainee.** The Royal College of Paediatrics and Child Health doesn't officially endorse sitting specialist exams during Foundation years and the Foundation programme actively discourages it (by not giving any study leave for exams, meaning that it all has to come out of your annual leave allowance). However, some people do choose to sit one, or sometimes two, of the written papers during their Foundation training. This shows your commitment to the specialty, which helps to improve your chances of gaining a place on a specialist paediatrics training programme. Passing at least one of the written papers as a Foundation trainee can really take off some of the pressure as a paediatric SHO. This not only helps the whole process to feel more relaxed but will also give you more freedom to take up other opportunities.

■ **Finding time for all the exams as a specialist trainee.** It is perfectly possible to fit all the exams into the first 3 years of training as long as you start early enough and don't have to take too many resits. There are three sittings of each exam every year, meaning that it is possible to have many separate attempts within a short space of time. Sitting exams as a specialist trainee means that you can apply for study leave in order to prepare for the exam and may have some financial support for attending revision courses.

■ **Rotations and rotas.** Rotations which are less demanding in terms of night and weekend shifts can be useful when studying for written exams as you will have more free time to do book work. Busy rotations at big general paediatric or tertiary paediatric units can be really useful when preparing for clinical exams as you will have the opportunity to see lots of children and work on your examination skills and see some rare pathology. If you have not yet applied for specialist training, it may be worth considering how you plan to fit in your exams when you are choosing which rotations you would like to do and at which stage.

■ **Finances**. Sitting exams is expensive, particularly if you have to sit some of the papers more than once. Try to budget for this when considering big expenses for the year. Given the financial as well as time implications, you should take each attempt seriously. Plan ahead, give yourself plenty of time to prepare and do lots of practice questions and any available practice papers.

■ **Talk to people who have recently passed the exams**. Talking to people who have passed recently can be really helpful in terms of taking their advice about how they prepared. It can also potentially save you a lot of money if they are willing to lend you the books that they used. If not, then trying the hospital library for books could also save you from shelling out extra money for these.

■ **Don't be disheartened**. The pass rate for professional postgraduate exams is much lower than for most medical school exams. Do not be disheartened if you do have to resit some of the papers and take the opportunity to learn from what happened. You will receive a breakdown of your marks for each of the topics on the paper so you can identify any problem areas and focus on those before your next attempt.

■ **Invest in practice questions**. There are lots of different versions available online and in book form. Practice questions are a great way of getting used to the style of questions and strategies in approaching the answer. They are also a great way of identifying topics which you need to do more reading on.

■ **Start with the hard bits**. The temptation with revision can be to start with topics you feel comfortable with and avoid the topics you don't like. Chances are, the topics you don't like are the ones you know least about and disciplining yourself to start with these can mean that you have plenty of time to learn and improve your knowledge in these areas.

■ **Do practice cases with senior colleagues**. When it comes to revising for your clinical exams, it is really important to get some feedback from your senior colleagues. Practising solely with your peers watching you can mean that you miss out on valuable feedback; they will not only have much less experience to offer but are also likely to be less critical, meaning that you miss out on the opportunity to improve. Find out if any of the consultants at your hospital are current clinical examiners and ask them if they would mind assessing you on some cases. You will be sent to a hospital outside your area for the clinical exam so these consultants will not be examining you on the day and their feedback can be enormously valuable in helping you to pass the exam.

How to boost your CV

Regardless of where you are in your career, there are some golden rules about making your CV look more impressive and setting yourself apart from the crowd.

■ Finish things. This can be easier said than done but so many people start pieces of work or projects which they don't finish. This is such a waste of your time and energy and may give you little or nothing to show for your efforts.

■ Don't overcommit. Think about how much time you have available before agreeing to take part in new things. Taking on too many projects at the same time means you are much less likely to finish any of them or to do them to a high standard. In order to avoid missing out on future opportunities, say yes but negotiate that the person asking does something for you in return, or agree to take on only a smaller portion of what they have asked for. If you do have to say no, make sure to tell them that you will do it another time but you are too busy at the moment.

■ Work with other people. Working on projects with colleagues means you can get through large volumes of work much more quickly and you all gain from the end result. It can also improve your team-working skills, which are highly sought after and should be mentioned at interviews.

■ Do what interests you. One way to ensure that your projects get finished and that you do them to a high standard is to choose something which interests you. Don't do something just because you think it will look good on your CV if the thought of doing it fills you with dread or boredom. Taking part in things which you find interesting or that you think are important will give you far more motivation to finish than scoring points alone.

■ Find people who inspire you. Inspiring and enthusiastic senior colleagues can help enormously, not just by offering you opportunities but with motivating you to take on new challenges and push yourself.

■ Update your CV. Whilst for many of the specialist programmes, you will need to fill in a generic application form, some deaneries may ask you to take a copy of your CV to interview with you and you may need to send it to people when other opportunities arise. Make sure you keep it up to date and keep it short. Previous achievements which were once significant will become less important as you progress so remember to go through and remove things as well as adding new achievements in. Keep the formatting clear and professional looking.

As well as this general advice on CV building, there are some specific things which you can do at different stages to set you apart from your peers and increase your chances of success.

CV building for medical students

This is an early stage to start thinking about your career but chances are, if you're reading this book, you're already pretty interested in a career in paediatrics. There are lots of things which you can do to find out more about the specialty to make sure it is the right choice for you. Also, because you have more time and energy than once you start working, this is a great time to complete projects which will look impressive later on.

Apply for Foundation posts in paediatrics

There are relatively few paediatric Foundation training jobs so this is not essential for being able to apply for paediatrics but it is certainly useful. This is a great time for you to test out how you feel about the actual job (which can sometimes be quite a different experience from doing a placement as a student) and will also help you to gain valuable insight for interview and lots of additional opportunities such as audits, improvement projects and teaching relevant to paediatrics. Think about the timing of the paediatric rotation so that you will have a chance to gain some experience prior to your applications for specialist training (which happen in the first rotation of FY2). If you don't manage to get a rotation in paediatrics as part of your Foundation years, you can always apply to do a taster week at a paediatric unit instead (see the CV Building for Foundation Trainees section below for more details). There is also now an attempt nationally to offer more rotations to Foundation trainees that involve working in the community setting or in psychiatry so try to get a rotation in community paediatrics or child and adolescent psychiatry if you can.

Special study modules and electives

Completing additional rotations in paediatrics as part of a special study module or during your medical elective can allow you to gain additional experience of paediatrics and help to demonstrate your interest in the specialty. There may even be an opportunity for you to take part in a small project or audit as part of the special study module which could be useful later on. Medical electives are a great time to gain an international perspective on child health and the challenges of high mortality rates in the under-5s in developing countries.

Prizes

There are numerous prizes available to medical students for accounts of interesting cases or essays on various subjects. For example, the Royal College of Paediatrics and Child Health runs a prize uniquely for medical students in addition to several prizes for which junior doctors and medical students are both eligible. These can look impressive on your CV and often also involve a financial reward.

Volunteer

Volunteering can be a hugely rewarding experience and a great way for you to learn new skills. There are so many different opportunities: helping with a play group for disabled children, working at a children's hospice or teaching sex education in schools. Look out for local and national children's charities which you can help with. The website www.do-it.org.uk allows you to search for volunteering opportunities in your local area by topic. Also, find out about any student initiatives at your university. Some of the following initiatives now have groups in medical schools. If there isn't one at your medical school already then contact them for help in setting up a local branch.

■ **Play4all**. This is a social enterprise set up by a medical student which aims to provide out-of-hours play facilities for children who are in hospital through medical students volunteering their time and skills (www.play4all.org.uk).

■ **Sexpression**. Medical students volunteer to provide informal sex and relationship sessions for young people to empower them to make informed decisions about their sexual health (www.sexpression.org.uk).

■ **Teddy Bear Hospital**. Medical students go into schools to teach young children about their health and about doctors and hospitals through play. The idea is to promote healthy lifestyles and also to prepare children so that visits to the doctor and hospital become less frightening.

Join or set up a paediatric society

Find out if your university already has a paediatric society and how to get involved. If there isn't one already, could you set one up yourself?

Attend a conference

There are national paediatric conferences held by undergraduates for undergraduates which you can attend. There are also student conferences in global health organised by Medsin, which include presentations and workshops on international child health (www.medsin.org). Medsin also oversee the international children's charity SKIP (Students for Kids International Projects) which supports child welfare in communities throughout the developing world. See the website www.skipkids.org.uk for details of how to get involved.

Become a medical student affiliate member of the RCPCH

You can become an affiliate member of the RCPCH as a medical student. It is free to become an affiliate member as a medical student but you can also choose to pay a (heavily subsidised) annual subscription for the journal *Archives of Disease in Childhood*. As an affiliate member you will get regular email updates from the Royal College, careers advice and access to members-only areas of the website and online publications. Go to www.rcpch.ac.uk/member-services to apply.

Additional qualifications

Many medical schools offer you the opportunity to complete an additional qualification such as a BSc. Consider choosing a BSc which is relevant to paediatrics, for example through the research project or essay topics which you choose.

CV building for Foundation trainees

Taster weeks

Don't worry if you have only recently considered paediatrics and don't have any Foundation jobs in the specialty; there are still opportunities to gain experience. During your Foundation training you can arrange a 'taster week' in a paediatric unit in order to learn more about the specialty and talk to paediatric trainees. Even if you have a Foundation job in paediatrics, you can apply to spend a taster week in community paediatrics or with the child and adolescent mental health team to gain further experience.

Careers events

The RCPCH runs careers events for Foundation doctors. Check the website for details or become a Foundation doctor affiliate member of the RCPCH to get regular updates about events.

Conferences

Attend paediatric conferences such as the RCPCH conference (which is an international conference) or your local paediatric deanery conference. This is a great way of learning about the latest developments in the specialty and hearing experts present their work. Try submitting an abstract of an audit or improvement project you have been involved in, as poster presentations at conferences look impressive on your CV.

Audits

Completing an audit is a compulsory part of Foundation training but you can make yourself stand out by going further than the basic requirements. Taking part in regular audits, leading audits yourself and completing the audit cycle (i.e. re-auditing after making a change) all help to highlight your motivation and ability to see a task through to completion. Presenting your findings at a regional or national meeting (as well as locally) looks impressive and gives you an opportunity to share your ideas with a wider audience. You can also submit an abstract of your audit findings to a conference or journal to gain credit by way of a poster or publication.

Exams

Sitting one of the paediatric MRCPCH exams during your Foundation years shows that you are committed to the specialty and can be useful when applying for specialist training.

Improvement projects

These can be challenging but rewarding to be involved in. Completion of an improvement project is also now a compulsory part of Foundation training so to stand out, you need to do more than the basics. Presenting your work at various patient safety or quality and improvement conferences is one way of helping to set you apart. There are also several places where you can try to get your work published such as *Casebook* (www.the-network.org.uk) and *BMJ Quality and Safety Journal.*

Life support training

Completion of a paediatric life support course can provide you with clinical skills for use during clinical placements (not just in paediatrics but in the emergency department or general practice). Completion of these courses also helps to set you apart from others by showing your commitment to pursuing a career in paediatrics.

Teaching and training in teaching

Teaching should be a standard part of all doctors' day-to-day work. Taking the initiative and setting up your own teaching programme to suit students' needs is impressive and if you can organise this regionally or across the entire medical school, this looks even better. Collecting feedback is important, as is being able to show how you've changed your teaching based on the feedback you've received from students. You may also find it useful to complete a training course in medical education. Many of these courses are available locally, sometimes free of charge for doctors working in teaching hospitals. Find out what is available at your trust and sign up early as they tend to be very popular.

CV building for specialist trainees

Subspecialties

You may already have an idea about whether or not you would like to sub-specialise within paediatrics. If you do think that you may apply for subspecialty training through the 'grid' process, it is worth trying to gain relevant experience to show your interest in the specialty. Try to get involved in audits or research in that area, apply for rotations in the earlier stages of your training which include time at a unit which specialises in your area of interest. Also, even if you know that you want to pursue the general paediatrics route, it is worth remembering that you can qualify as a general paediatrician with a specialist interest. This means that you have more opportunity to pursue areas which interest you without having to commit solely to that subspecialty. It can also be helpful when applying for consultant jobs to have a specialist interest which you can add to the department.

Out of programme (OOP)

It is possible to take time 'out of programme' for a variety of different reasons. Each of these needs approval from the Royal College and your deanery to go ahead and the national guidance on OOP time is outlined in the 'Gold Guide' (the postgraduate training guide produced by Modernising Medical Careers). The different OOP opportunities are as follows.

■ **Out of Programme Clinical Training (OOPT)**. You can apply to the General Medical Council for approval of pursuing training abroad for a year, which will contribute towards your overall training (i.e. you will still progress a year within the training programme).

■ **Out of Programme Experience (OOPE)**. This is for cases which do not receive approval from the GMC as a training post. This means that you can pursue training abroad but the year will not count towards your specialist training and when you return, you will continue training at the same point as you left.

■ **Out of Programme Research (OOPR)**. This allows time to pursue research and it is possible to have the time approved by the GMC so that it counts towards your specialty training. This research is usually undertaken as part of a higher qualification such as a PhD or MSc.

■ **Out of Programme Career Break (OOPC)**. This can be time out for maternity leave or childcare responsibilities or because of your own or a family member's ill health.

Most people use the term 'ooo-pee' (OOPE) when referring to any of the above four variations of time out of programme. For more information look at the 'Gold Guide' which can be downloaded from www.mmc.nhs.uk.

Further qualifications

You don't necessarily have to take time out of programme to study for post-graduate qualifications. There are flexible Master's and diploma courses which can be completed over an extended period of time rather than as a full-time year-long course. You could consider pursuing an additional qualification in medical education or a Master's in international child health. There are lots of different courses available.

Clinical governance – more than just audit

It is important to undertake audits to make sure that the care we provide for patients lives up to the expected standards. Sadly, audit is frequently treated as a tick box exercise rather than something which can have a positive impact on patient care. This is partly because many junior doctors just complete audits which their senior colleagues have told them to do and have no interest in the subject themselves. This can mean that they take on something too big for them to realistically complete and the audit feels like a tedious task which drags on for an extended period of time. As a consequence, many people start audits which they don't subsequently finish and therefore waste a lot of time and energy on work which they receive no credit for and the patients receive no benefit from.

If you are going to complete an audit then try to pick the topic yourself and choose something small which you can realistically complete. Remember

 Top Tip

Choose something which you feel strongly about or are interested in as the topic of your audit or improvement project. You are far more likely to see it through to completion and make it a success if you care about the outcome.

that audits are only useful if something changes as a result of what you have found out. Many people do the data collection and analysis bit, present a list of recommendations and then think that the audit is done. But if you want to have any impact on patient care then you need to make sure that these recommendations become real-life changes. Also, if you manage to put some changes in place then there is an opportunity to *re-audit* and see if there has been any improvement following your intervention. This is what people mean when they refer to 'closing the loop' with an audit. Not only is this far more satisfying as you can see a change in practice resulting from your interventions but it will also gain you far more credit when it comes to building an impressive CV for job applications. Doctors who have taken part in a complete audit cycle (i.e. audit, change something, re-audit) are rare and this can really make you stand out at interview.

Service improvement projects

Audit is the process of comparing practice in your hospital or department with a recognised minimum standard and seeing whether or not you meet it. But what if there is no agreed standard? What if the problems you notice aren't clinical ones but to do with the processes and systems in place within the hospital? What if you want to find ways to provide excellent care, not just meet a minimum standard?

This is where service improvement projects or quality improvement projects feature. You may hear people talking about a 'quip'; what they are referring to is a QIP or quality improvement project. The idea of having such projects run by junior doctors and medical students has become popular over the last few years as people have realised that they often have the enthusiasm, determination and insight to make real differences to the quality of service provided for patients.

Completing a service improvement project can be a much more rewarding experience than half-doing an audit and not implementing any change as a result. Junior doctors have a unique insight into the day-to-day running of the health service and can have a large and positive impact if they choose to change some of the things that they see going wrong. In fact, completion of a service improvement project now forms part of the curriculum for FY2 doctors (Academy of Medical Royal Colleges Foundation Programme Committee 2012).

Find something which annoys you or that just doesn't work properly for staff, patients or their relatives and try to think of a better way of doing it. This can be great fun as it is a chance for you to be creative in coming up with innovative solutions to problems. Here are some suggestions for how to make sure your service improvement project is a success.

■ **Work in a team**. This not only has the possibility to make the whole experience much more enjoyable but also means that you can maintain momentum for the project as it is unlikely that you are all going to be on night shifts or annual leave at the same time so there is someone there to help keep the ball rolling.

■ **Have other professionals working as part of your team**. Don't just get together a group of doctors as you will end up with a rather one-dimensional view of the problem. A team which includes lots of different professionals (e.g. a nurse, a pharmacist, an occupational therapist and a junior doctor) can be a much more powerful combination. Your different experiences and backgrounds can bring real strength to the team and ultimately to the project you are trying to complete.

■ **Think small**. Given the frequency with which we all rotate through different jobs and between different hospitals, it can be difficult to find time to finish off a project before having to move on to a new trust. By focusing on a much smaller scale project to start with, you can see some of the results of your efforts and help to iron out any initial problems.

■ **Collect evidence**. Sometimes it is obvious to you that something isn't working or it seems like common sense that it would be better to do things another way. However, there are lots of other people whom you need to persuade, many of whom will have a totally different perspective on things. This is why you need some objective evidence to use to persuade people that the change is needed and afterwards, that the change has worked. Things like staff and patient surveys or some kind of measurement of time or cost savings can give you some numbers to back up what you are saying.

■ Learn from previous examples.

It may be that someone elsewhere has already had a similar idea and you can build on what they learnt from the process and point to their successes as an example of how things could be improved in your own hospital. The Network (www.the-network.org.uk) is an online resource of service improvement projects and audits. It also produces a journal called *Casebook* to which you can submit an abstract of your project once completed. The BMJ Quality Improvement Reports is an online searchable archive of improvement projects (http://qir.bmj.com). It contains projects submitted by junior doctors who have subscribed to BMJ Quality Improvement Programmes (but you do not need a subscription to read the reports) which is an online tool to guide you through the quality improvement process, including helping to match you with a consultant mentor (http://quality.bmj.com). Many trusts now run their own quality improvement programmes for junior doctors. Find out if there is one in your area as they may provide support for your project and have records of previous projects run by others in your area.

■ Make it sustainable. It's all very

well to come up with a fantastic new system but if the whole thing falls apart when you're not there then it isn't of any lasting use. Creating a change which is sustainable is really hard so do spend time thinking about how you can ensure that everything runs smoothly without you there overseeing it. This is another reason why having a multidisciplinary team can be such an advantage as other professionals may be permanent staff at that hospital and can help ensure that the changes continue after you've left.

■ Engage your stakeholders. This is

fancy management jargon for getting the right people on your side. Whenever you're hoping to change something, you need to think about who and what those changes are going to affect and how. Who are you relying on for the change to happen? Who could potentially obstruct the whole project? What crucial pieces of equipment need to be available? This is about thinking through who the people with power and authority are. In some cases authority and power are not necessarily held by the same person. For example, a senior manager at the hospital will have the authority to agree to, or refuse, certain things which you propose but they may hold relatively little power in ensuring that the day-to-day running of your project goes smoothly. By contrast, the hospital porters, who have relatively little authority, actually hold a lot of power in some cases. If you have a new idea for the way that blood specimens are processed but the porters are not happy with, or not aware of, how you want to alter the way in which they work then the whole project can fail. Spend plenty of time working out who your stakeholders are and even more time holding meetings for them, sending out emails, producing posters and surveys to find out what they think of your ideas and then adapt it based on their suggestions. This can be a lengthy process and a trying one at times.

■ **Be patient**. Once you dig below the surface of what seemed a relatively simple problem, you often find all sorts of other complex processes are involved. It can be exasperating sometimes finding

out about various rules and processes which appear to be inefficient or pointless and sometimes it can feel as if people are being deliberately obstructive. The important thing is to try to remain patient and if email or phone communication isn't working, arrange a meeting face to face as this can sometimes make a world of difference. Try to understand where the other person is coming from and their reservations as fully as you can. This will help you to find ways of getting that person on board and may make your final project much more successful as a result. They may have spotted a potential pitfall that you hadn't seen, so try to view their criticism as constructive feedback to help make the service even better.

 Top Tip

Whether you have taken part in an audit or a service improvement project, the important thing is to complete it and to present and publish your results. There will be many local meetings you can present at (grand rounds, departmental meetings) but try to present your findings more widely than this in order to make it look more impressive on your CV. Asking for a slot to speak at a regional meeting can be a good start and submit your work as a poster or presentation for a conference (an international one is best but national ones are good too). There are many patient safety and quality care conferences (including international ones) where you can present your work. Submit your findings to be published in a peer-reviewed journal too, even if it is in the form of a short 'letter to the editor'.

Patient safety

Patient safety has become a much more prominent topic over the past few years with many junior doctors taking part in projects and contributing to a shift in culture. Safety processes are engrained in the day-to-day working of high-risk industries such as offshore oil rigs and the airline industry because small human errors in these settings can cost lives. Given the obvious parallels, it may seem odd that such safety systems and human error training are much less widespread in clinical medicine. However, in recent years there has been increasing interest from the medical profession in what lessons can be learned from the way in which the airline industry functions in order to improve patient safety. This is in part thanks to the work of Martin Bromiley, an airline pilot whose wife died as a result of medical error, who established the Clincial Human Factors Group (CHFG) (www.chfg.org). The CHFG runs frequent seminars for medical professionals and its aim is to promote safer, higher quality healthcare by increasing awareness of human factors and how to prevent human error becoming an actual harm to a patient. A moving and thought-provoking video about the errors which lead to Mrs Bromiley's death, called 'Just a routine operation', can be found on the CHFG website.

If you have any doubts about the importance of patient safety then take a look at the patient stories website (www.patientstories.org.uk). It tells the stories of patients whose lives have been lost or otherwise affected as a result of medical error and analyses some of the lessons which can be learned by the medical profession from these examples.

Less than full-time training

At some stage in your training you may have other things which you need to dedicate time to as well as your clinical practice. This may be taking a more active role in research or delivery of teaching or having more time available for personal reasons such as caring for your own children or relatives. Less than full-time training is well established within paediatrics (as a specialty it

Top Tip

If you are working less than full time, you may be entitled to pay reduced rate subscription fees to the RCPCH, General Medical Council, British Medical Association and your defence union (MPS or MDU). More information about this can be found on the RCPCH website.

pioneered many of the flexible training arrangements) and there are now agreed national guidelines on the subject from the General Medical Council and the NHS. Copies of the relevant guidance can be found on the RCPCH website along with lots of other information.

Each region has its own named consultant representatives who co-ordinate less than full-time training and many places will also have a trainee committee to provide support, information and advice for trainees who are working less than full time. There is useful information and advice available in the postgraduate doctors section on the Medical Careers website (www.medicalcareers.nhs.uk).

Some things to be aware of if you are considering working less than full time include the following.

■ **Money**. Working less than full time means that your salary will be reduced in proportion to the hours that you work. There is national guidance on how salaries for part-time workers are calculated which can allow you to work out how much you will be paid if you know the full basic salary for that job. This document, 'Equitable Pay', is available to download from the less than full-time page of the RCPCH website.

■ **Application process**. If you are hoping to reduce your working hours then you need to let the deanery know at least 3 months in advance so it can make the appropriate arrangements for service provision and funding. It may help to discuss it first with your educational supervisor or one of the named consultant representatives for your area (whose names and email addresses are available on the RCPCH website on the less than full-time training page). Less than full-time training can be done in several different ways but the one which tends to be most popular with deaneries and hospitals is the job-sharing option. This requires you to find someone who is willing to share a full-time post with you and to agree on how you split the hours. This can be a lengthy and time-consuming process so allow yourself plenty of time to sort out all the paperwork.

■ **Delaying becoming a consultant**. Becoming a consultant requires you to be awarded a Certificate of Completion of Training (CCT). Although there is now emphasis on competency-based assessment of whether or not you can progress (instead of simply spending the required amount of time doing the job), your predicted CCT date will be delayed as a result of part-time training as you will not be able to gain the same experience in the same timeframe as your full-time colleagues.

■ **Time**. The General Medical Council dictates that the minimum amount a *trainee* is allowed to work is 50% of full time (although this can be negotiated in exceptional circumstances). This is because otherwise your training would take an enormously long time to complete and less time than this may affect the quality of your work. You can work much less than this but it will not count towards your training. For example, you may have a year out of programme but want to work one day a week of clinical work during this time to help to maintain your skills. *For more about out of programme opportunities see the CV Building for Specialist Trainees section above.*

■ **Peer group**. Training less than full time can sometimes make you feel that you don't have a peer group in the same way as full-time trainees do. You may find that you miss the camaraderie of group who are doing exams and interviews at the same time as you. One way to find more consistency may be to join the less than full-time trainee committee where you will find others in a similar situation and be able to influence deanery policy in relation to less than full-time training.

■ **Education**. It can be difficult to keep up to date with your skills and gain adequate learning opportunities when you are working less than full time. Make sure that you put yourself forward for opportunities when they arise as you are just as entitled to learn as your full-time colleagues and have less time in which to do it. Going back to work after a period of non-clinical work may feel daunting and arranging 'keep in touch' days during periods of prolonged leave can be helpful for keeping up with the latest training. Some deaneries also offer 'return to work' refresher courses.

Teaching and training

There are lots of opportunities to get involved in teaching at all stages; even as a medical student, you can teach those in year groups below you and your peers. Don't forget that you can very usefully get involved in teaching across the disciplines too and help with teaching student nurses and allied health professionals.

Things to consider when teaching include the following.

■ **Plan ahead if possible**. In most cases you should know about your teaching commitments beforehand so taking the time to plan the session can make your teaching much more effective. Work out what key learning points you want students to take away from the session, think about how much time you will spend on each topic or activity and prepare any necessary materials (e.g. slideshow and handouts for lectures, copies of case studies for small group teaching, a whiteboard and pens that work).

■ **Less is more**. Avoid the temptation to cram too much into your teaching sessions. This can make them feel rushed or chaotic and you may overrun, meaning that you have to abandon the session before the end if you or the students have other commitments. Think realistically about how much time it will take to go through certain activities or talking through certain topics and then allow a

bit extra on top of this. If you know how long you've allowed for each bit, you can keep an eye on the time during the session and keep things moving along at an appropriate pace.

■ **Know your audience**. It is really important to know who you are teaching and what they already know in order to make it useful for them. On a basic level, you can find out which year group students or trainees belong to in order to gain a rough idea of how much they are likely to know already. There can be a wide variation in the previous experience and knowledge of students and doctors who are working at the same level. Asking at the beginning of the session specific questions about what people already know will allow you to tailor your session to the group as best you can. Don't panic if one of them has done a PhD on the topic you're about to teach. It is far better to establish this at the beginning and to make use of their expertise in the teaching session.

■ **Make it relevant**. When you are investigating who you will be teaching, you should find out what they will need or want to know. Are there any exams coming up for them soon? Is there a curriculum or a list of competencies which they are required to meet? Knowing about this means you can pitch your teaching sessions at the right level and cover the relevant topics.

■ **Don't be afraid to change the plan**. Even if you have planned a session down to the last detail, things can happen to disrupt it. The students may not be able to work through problems as quickly as you'd anticipated or need clarification on a certain issue before they are able to move on. If this happens and you find that you are overrunning, you may need to miss out something you were planning to cover in order to make sure that the session still runs to time.

■ **Involve the patient**. If you are doing bedside teaching, you should talk to children and their families beforehand to check that they are happy to participate. Giving the patient and their family members an active role in the teaching session is a much more empowering experience for them and allows students to learn more than they could from a textbook or a lecture from you. Patients with long-term conditions and their families often become experts and may have more specialist knowledge than you do on certain aspects so make good use of this. Make sure that you go back after the teaching session in case the child or their family members have any questions as a result of the teaching session.

■ **Be punctual and enthusiastic**. It is understandable that sometimes clinical emergencies arise which prevent you from attending a planned teaching session but this should be very much an exception. Turn up on time and call ahead if you know that you will be unavoidably late. It is basic courtesy for the people you are teaching and it doesn't set up the session well if you are late or appear as if the teaching session is just an inconvenience to you. If you know in advance about a teaching session then arrange appropriate cover for the time which you are going to be away from clinical duties and get someone to hold your bleep for you.

■ **Collect feedback**. A key way of improving the quality of your teaching is to find out what students actually think of it. You can do this in many ways and be creative about how you go about it (it doesn't always have to be a paper form at the end of the session). Think about what information you actually want to find out from students and ask specific questions which will allow you to gain constructive feedback. It can also be very valuable to gain feedback from a colleague on your teaching. This can be one of your peers but it can be particularly helpful if you ask a senior colleague with lots of teaching experience. They will be able to offer you more specific and constructive feedback than it is possible to gain from student evaluation forms. Don't forget that you have to complete a supervised learning event on 'developing the clinical teacher' and this can be an ideal opportunity to complete one of these. More information on WORK-BASED ASSESSMENTS and SUPERVISED LEARNING EVENTS below.

■ **Additional qualifications**. Given that teaching in a school requires lots of training in how to educate, it does seem surprising that often doctors will receive no training at all before being expected to teach. Attending training sessions to gain some basic understanding of how to structure your teaching effectively, how adults learn, how to make the most of different forms of teaching can really help to get you started and gain confidence. There are many courses available, some of which may even be offered for free by medical schools to doctors working in teaching hospitals. Check with your local medical education team or medical school to find out more. If you are keen to do a lot of teaching, you may wish to consider studying for a formal qualification in medical education such as a diploma or take time out of programme to work as a fellow in medical education.

Work-based assessments and e-portfolios

Work-based assessments and e-portfolios are now included in all levels of training (and at many medical schools). WORK-BASED ASSESSMENTS are also sometimes known as SUPERVISED LEARNING EVENTS. Trying to make sure that you get everything done can feel really tedious at times and people often end up treating it as a 'tick-box exercise'. However, if used properly, you can turn them into helpful experiences for your learning. You'll have to complete them either way so you might as well try to make them useful rather than feeling like a tedious waste of time. Here are some top tips for how to get the most out of work-based assessments.

■ **Don't leave it until the last minute**. If you space your work-based assessments evenly throughout your placement, this gives you an opportunity to ask for feedback from people you have worked with and allows you to keep an eye on your progress and identify things you need to work on. Also, given that many people do leave

completion of their assessment to the last minute, the registrars and consultants you ask will probably have been inundated with requests from other trainees, meaning that they may not have time to give you proper feedback or even to fill in your assessment at all.

■ **Don't request an assessment several weeks after it happened**. Ideally you should try to fill in your assessments at the time but this is rarely possible and often you need to send an electronic request or 'ticket' to the person who you want to complete an assessment for you. This means that you need their email address so make sure to note it down. Make a point of sending the ticket as soon as possible after the assessment has happened (the same day if possible) because if you forget and end up sending a request several weeks later, you can guarantee that the person doing your assessment will have forgotten all about the details!

■ **Ask the assessor what works best for them**. Don't assume that all assessors will want you to email them an electronic request. Some may find it easier to fill it in there and then or others may ask if they can meet you at a later date to fill it in with them (sometimes because they want you to guide them through using the computer program). Make sure to ask what they would like to increase the chances of them completing the assessment for you.

■ **Give the assessor some information about the case**. Obviously, don't use any confidential information about the patient but a quick summary can help remind your assessor which case you want them to assess, e.g. 4-year-old boy seen in A&E with shortness of breath, we discussed my history and examination findings and initial management plan.

■ **Little and often**. Trying to keep on top of your e-portfolio by doing little bits frequently feels so much better than neglecting it all year and then having to give up an entire weekend to sort it out. You won't pass your year unless the e-portfolio is up to date and evidence from your e-portfolio may be requested at interviews so make sure that it is of high quality.

■ **Choose a good time**. Finding the right opportunities to get your assessments done helps to make them more meaningful and useful for you and increases the chances of you getting all of them completed. Quiet night shifts can sometimes be good times to do a quick work-based assessment as with the lower burden of administrative work, your job is more clinically based and sometimes you will be working in a team with the registrar. Here are some suggestions for the different assessments.

– **Case-based discussions (CBDs)** can be easily completed during on-call shifts when you will be presenting a summary of the cases you have seen to the registrar or consultant anyway at some point. Asking them beforehand if they would mind doing one as a case-based discussion can be an efficient way of getting assessments done which saves time for both of you and is useful as you will get immediate feedback on how you have managed a case.

– **Mini clinical evaluation exercises (mini-CEXs)** can sometimes be done on the ward round. Ask the person running the ward round if they would mind if you examine one of the patients whilst they observe. This can be an efficient use of time rather than having to engineer separate situations.

– **Directly observed procedural skills (DOPS)** can also be filled in by senior nursing staff who are trained in the procedure, so if a nurse has been helping you to put in a cannula, you can try asking them to complete a DOPS for you.

– **Reflections** are much quicker and easier to do if you complete them at the time and will also be much more useful for you as an exercise. This can be a really constructive way of improving your practice if done properly. Try to complete reflections the same evening or at least the same week as the event you are reflecting on. *For more about reflective writing see Chapter 10 – Looking After Yourself.*

– **Developing the clinical teacher assessment**. An ideal opportunity to ask an assessor to fill one of these in is following a presentation you have done at an audit meeting, journal club or grand round.

Useful websites

Royal College of Paediatrics and Child Health: www.rcpch.ac.uk. This website has all the information you need about the specialist training structure, application processes and exams as well child health guidelines and reports.

NHS Institute for Innovation and Improvement: www.institute.nhs.uk This website has loads of great learning resources on patient safety, quality and value and innovation.

The Network: www.the-network.org.uk. This is an online collection of service improvement projects and audits which you can search through to look for interesting projects others have done. It publishes a journal called *Casebook*.

Patient stories: www.patientstories.org.uk. This is a website set up by the friends and relatives of patients who have lost their lives as a result of medical error in an attempt to help doctors to learn from what happened and prevent similar events from happening in the future.

Patient Safety First: www.patientsafetyfirst. nhs.uk. This was a campaign run within the NHS and although the campaign itself has now finished, the website remains as an excellent resource for learning more about patient safety.

BMJ Quality Improvement Reports: http://qir. bmj.com. This is an online searchable archive of improvement projects. It contains projects submitted by junior doctors who have subscribed to BMJ Quality Improvement Programmes (but you do not need a subscription to read the reports).

BMJ Quality Improvement Programmes: http://quality.bmj.com. This is an online tool to guide you through the quality improvement process, including helping to match you with a consultant mentor, learning modules and templates to guide you through how to approach the project.

Clinical Human Factors Group: www.chfg.org. Find out more about human factors and how knowledge of this can be used to minimise risks to patient safety.

Institute for Healthcare Improvement: www.ihi.org. This website has lots of useful learning material relating to quality improvement in healthcare with case studies and examples of other people's projects.

Medical Careers: www.medicalcareers.nhs.uk. Lots of information about the different stages of medical training.

References

Academy of Medical Royal Colleges Foundation Programme Committee (2012) *The UK Foundation Programme Curriculum*. Academy of Medical Royal Colleges, London.

Royal College of Paediatrics and Child Health (2013) *The Royal College of Paediatrics and Child Health Trainees' Guide to Training in Research for the Benefit of Children*. Royal College of Paediatrics and Child Health, London.

Index

Page numbers in *italics* denote figures, those in **bold** denote tables.

The Hands-on Guide to Practical Paediatrics, First Edition. Rebecca Hewitson and Caroline Fertleman.
© 2014 John Wiley & Sons, Ltd. Published 2014 by John Wiley & Sons, Ltd.
Companion Website: www.wileyhandsonguides.com/paediatrics